AAHA's Complete Guide for the
Veterinary Client Service Representative

AAHA's Complete Guide FOR THE
VETERINARY
Client Service Representative

JILL RENFREW, MBA, CVPM, ACC

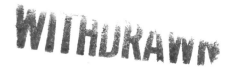

AAHA
press

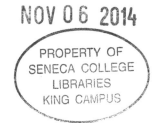

American Animal Hospital Association Press
12575 West Bayaud Avenue
Lakewood, Colorado 80228
800-883-6301
press.aahanet.org

ISBN 13: 978-1-58326-192-7

Library of Congress Cataloging-in-Publication Data

Renfrew, Jill.

AAHA's complete guide for the veterinary client service representative / Jill Renfrew.

  p. ; cm.

  Complete guide for the veterinary client service representative

  Includes bibliographical references.

  ISBN 978-1-58326-192-7

  I. American Animal Hospital Association. II. Title. III. Title: Complete guide for the veterinary

    client service representative.

  [DNLM: 1. Veterinary Medicine--organization & administration. 2. Hospitals, Animal--organization

  & administration. 3. Interpersonal Relations. 4. Practice Management--organization &

  administration. SF 745]

  SF604.6

  636.08'321068--dc23

                                                                    2013011639

Developmental Edit: Bess Maher
Interior Design: Erin Farrell / Factor E Creative
Cover Design: Robin Baker

Dedication

This text is dedicated to veterinary managerial professionals who desire the best for and from their team, who understand their integral role in supporting the human–animal bond, and who have a big-picture view of their managerial responsibilities and a strong desire to augment veterinarians' drive for superior health care with their own personal drive for excellence.

It is also dedicated to the client service representatives who, in their own words, "are the first contact for clients, inspire trust and confidence, set the tone for the client's visit, and develop client–receptionist partnerships" in the provision of quality pet health care.

Special thanks to Sharon Finster, DVM, DACVECC, and Dawn Fiedorczyk, DVM, for help with the common emergencies and vaccination schedule sections of this text.

TABLE OF CONTENTS

TO THE MANAGER

If you are reading this, you are looking for a more complete method for training your client service representative (CSR). Perhaps you have previously used an on-the-job training program or a combination of a phase training task list and on-the-job training time. Although either will teach your new team member the tasks that he needs to accomplish, it will not impart the additional CSI (client service intelligence) that is necessary to perform well in this position.

As you know, the veterinary business environment has changed dramatically. Our clients are knowledgeable and savvy. They demand excellent service and want their needs met in a friendly, efficient manner, and if their needs aren't met, they aren't afraid to use social media to post reviews of their experiences. When we turn a new CSR out into that environment without proper training, we are setting him up for defeat and ourselves up for headaches of migraine intensity.

You also know how difficult it is to find high-quality CSRs. Many of us are turning to individuals who have their initial training outside the veterinary profession in hospitality or other service professions. Whether he comes from outside or inside the veterinary industry, we know that we must make the new team member feel that he fits in and help him understand his role in the practice at large in order to create a valuable team player. We must inspire him as well as train him.

An essential part of integrating new individuals to the team is helping them absorb a big-picture view of your practice. This book is designed to bridge your needs for tasks such as training and the necessity of creating a better understanding of the CSR's role in the practice. It includes specific task instruction and standard operating procedures (SOPs) while inviting your new team member to see his role in providing excellent pet care and contributing to the practice's success. We recommend that you read through the text to ensure that the SOPs match those of your practice. The accompanying CD format for the text makes the content entirely customizable. Because every practice is unique, there will undoubtedly be sections, especially the SOPs, you will want to customize for your new employee.

Managing People

People have different behavioral characteristics. You may have heard of the Myers-Briggs Type Indicator[1] or the DISC[2] behavioral characteristic assessments used by many human resources professionals. These assessments are designed to help you better understand the characteristics displayed by your individual team members and can be helpful in understanding what makes a team member tick. Although a full explanation of these assessments is beyond the scope of this text, in general, using behavioral characteristic assessments allows us to evaluate how an individual acts and performs in a particular situation and to extrapolate that information to ascertain common characteristics. Many assessments categorize individuals into groups with characteristics such as extroversion/introversion, dominant/submissive, thinking/feeling, and compliant/independent. Knowing something about an individual's behavioral "type" can allow you to customize the learning experience. We recommend that you investigate using behavioral assessments for your team and cultivate an understanding of this information to enhance your management ability.

It is also important to remember that people have different learning styles. Experts in organizational learning and behavioral psychology have developed many theories of how people learn and the best methods with which to teach them new information. It is a good idea to familiarize yourself with these theories and to recognize the importance of including aspects of each learning style in your training program. In general, you should be reaching out to new team members with learning challenges that work for all types of learners by designing your training program to include several learning style components. As you develop your training program, you may want to keep some of the following methods in mind.

Use All the Senses

Some individuals learn better by reading information, others when they hear information related to them, and still others by actually performing the tasks. When instructing a new team member, offer as many of these types of learning opportunities as the information will allow.

Set and Review Goals

There is an old adage that if you set no goals, you are sure to achieve them. Know yourself, and let your new team member know just what you are requiring of him in each new task and situation. It is a good idea to have these goals as part of the written training program so everyone knows where they are headed.

Use Positive Feedback and Reinforcement

The task of training is closely associated with coaching your new team member. Offering encouragement creates an environment in which the new team member feels safe enough to ask questions when they arise and try new things when the situation requires. As a general rule, try to keep the positive feedback about performance of new tasks at a five-to-one ratio: five positive comments to one negative one. Some management professionals report that it takes five positive comments to outweigh one negative comment.

Vary the Focus

Give the new team member information about the importance of the components of the task and its importance in the overall function of your practice. Some team members understand a task and are motivated to perform well because they like getting all the details right; others find their motivation in understanding the big picture.

The Importance of Coaching

The veterinary culture can be hard on new team members. The physical veterinary office environment can be stressful and the learning environment pressured. Training time and resources are limited. Sometimes it seems that longtime team members have forgotten what it is like to be new. They expect quick assimilation of information and critical thinking that are beyond a new team member's frame of reference. As a manager, remember to slow down and remind others of the overwhelming amount of information involved with learning your practice's processes and procedures. Brief longtime team members on their role in the learning process and choose appropriate team members to mentor new individuals. Use a training checklist so that everyone knows what is required of them in the process and so the new team member's progress is readily apparent for review. We all need to embrace the concept of protecting, challenging, and coaching the new trainee.

It is important for managers to understand their own behavioral characteristics and actively pursue expanding these to meet an individual team member's needs. For an example, although you may be a direct and decisive personality, as many managers are, your trainee may be introverted and introspective. You may like short direct conversations that dump information from one vessel to another. Your trainee may be too scared by your approach to learn the information you are presenting. He may need a more indirect method of assimilating new information accompanied by much encouragement. Coaching involves slowing down and allowing the learning process to be as important as the outcome. Remember to follow the positive enforcement rule and ask for feedback on how you are doing to meet the new team member's needs as well as how he is adapting to his new environment. Frequent give-and-take conversations help the trainee know where he stands in the training process.

The Importance of a Job Description and Training Schedule

Starting a new job is confusing and overwhelming. When we ask a new team member to learn processes and procedures without a description of what is expected and a timeline for improvement, it is like asking him to take a trip across country without a map. Progress will be slow and accompanied by several wrong turns. Take the time to create a thorough job description and a timeline for the new CSR. A good job description defines the new hire's tasks and how those tasks are integral to the practice. Together, these two documents will help you define just what the job entails and let the new CSR know what you expect of him. You will achieve better results from training when these two components are used in the process.

The Process of On-boarding

On-boarding is a human resources phrase that describes the process of assimilating a new team member into your practice. It refers to the process that your new employee experiences while acclimating to your practice and includes all of his experiences, what he needs to know, the skills that he needs to acquire, and the cultural norms he needs to understand in order to perform his duties and feel like he belongs in the practice.

On-boarding should cover everything from the client service job description to real-time shift responsibilities. Presenting the new team member with a good job description is the best way to start the on-boarding process. This should be followed by a thorough orientation to the facility and an overview of the practice's culture, processes, and team structure. The training timeline should be introduced and thoroughly reviewed with the new team member. He should be provided with a copy of the timeline in order to track his own progress. Assigning trainers and mentors from the team will help bond the new individual and encourage him to ask the many questions that come up during the training process. Frequent check-in meetings—allowing the new team member to review what he has already learned and focus on what is to come—are very helpful. The process your practice uses to provide the new team member with feedback on his training progress should be defined so he knows what to expect. For instance, a new team member will want to know whether you will meet with him weekly for a cumulative review or provide feedback at the moment he makes an error.

An SOP for on-boarding is included in Appendix B and is customizable to your practice.

Putting It All Together for Your New Employee

We must nurture a good fit. This text assumes that you have done your homework during the hiring process and that you believe the new team member has potential for success within your practice. The rest of the story remains for you to orchestrate. You and your team must create an overall culture where learning is facilitated. You must create a learning organization driven by the core values, mission, and vision statements of the practice (see Chapter 1), understanding and encouraging individual differences, and where mastery of skills and tasks is approached as the responsibility of the collective team. The individual job categories in your veterinary practice include varied functions within the whole culture and system. Unifying them into a cohesive organization is your role and responsibility. It begins by creating an appropriate learning environment for each new team member. This CSR manual is designed to help you with one small part of that overall goal: creating a professional, knowledgeable, and savvy client service team.

How to Use This Manual

The manual comes with a CD that contains a Word document of the full contents. The print version includes information that will not be specific to your practice, such as a mission statement and SOPs. Each time the manual mentions something that would benefit from customization, a graphic of a pencil and paper will appear. This will tell you and your employees that the information does not reflect the way you do things at your practice but rather one recommended way of doing things. To avoid that, you can customize the CD version, which will also have these graphics. You can delete the graphics and the text that requires customization and type in the pertinent information. If you haven't established all your protocols, this may require effort on the part of a small leadership team. You may also want your front-office team to weigh in on the hospital information and procedures. The manager's appendix, Appendix B, contains more information about the customizable material, so when you see the ✎ graphic, you can turn to it for additional information before customizing your manual, although not all the customizable material is discussed at length there.

TO THE NEW TEAM MEMBER

Every veterinary hospital is unique and our practice has specific characteristics, processes, and idiosyncrasies that make us special. We want you to know and understand who we are and how we work together. We value what you can bring to the group and invite you to become an essential part of the team as we work together to provide excellent service to our clients and high-quality health care to their pets.

Our History

Welcome Aboard!

Thanks for joining our team. We hope that you will find your professional experience with us exciting and rewarding. We are providing you with this manual by way of introduction to our profession, our practice, and your responsibilities. We want you to know that we will support you as you learn your new tasks. We welcome your feedback on the process and ask that you approach us directly with any concerns that arise during your training. You will have a direct supervisor and be assigned other mentoring teammates. We will provide you with an organizational chart with a bird's-eye view of the organizational structure of our practice. It shows the flow of responsibility and oversight within our hospital. We wish you the best during your training process.

You have been given a copy of our employee handbook. The information contained there will be important for you during your time with our hospital. It will provide information on our standard employment policies that will affect you. It is your responsibility to understand and comply with the information in that text. If you have any questions about it, please ask your supervisor.

How to Use This Manual

Each time the manual mentions something that requires customization, a graphic of a pencil and paper will appear. This will tell you that the information in the manual does not necessarily reflect the way in which you do things at your practice but is simply one recommended way of doing things. Your manager may have an electronic version of this manual that includes your practice-specific information. However, much of the information in this text is general and is pertinent to any veterinary practice.

SOPs have been included and may have been customized by your practice. These are designed to give you a clear, concise explanation of how certain things are done at your practice. When you encounter an SOP, read it carefully and ask questions of your supervisor or trainer until you understand and can perform the processes and procedures it outlines.

CHAPTER ONE

So You Are New Here!

So you are new here! Our veterinary practice offers new team members an opportunity to become an integral part of the lives of our clients and patients as you assimilate into our culture, become familiar with our processes, and acquaint yourself with veterinary medicine. Our CSRs are vital to our practice of medicine and to our business success. This introductory chapter is designed to give you an overview of the underlying principles of your employment with us. We hope that you are excited to join us!

OUR HOSPITAL'S CORE VALUES, MISSION, AND VISION

Each of us lives by a set of values that we have developed over time. Our values define who we are and how we go about our daily tasks. Although we don't think about these things, they help us make decisions every day. They include such concepts as honesty, hard work, the importance of family, and financial security. Our practice has developed a set of these core values as well. We live by them, and they influence every decision that we make together. Many practices find that values like the following help them make good daily decisions at work:

- **Animal welfare.** We believe in the value of the profession of veterinary medicine.
- **Promoting the human–animal bond.** We believe that pets and people share a special bond.
- **Quality.** We believe that pets and their owners deserve high-quality pet health care.
- **Compassion.** We will care for our clients, for their pets, and for each other.
- **Teamwork.** We believe that we are stronger and better as we work together.
- **Respect.** We believe that every person and pet deserves proper respect.
- **Honesty.** We believe in telling the truth.

- **Responsibility.** We recognize our individual and collective responsibilities to the clients and pets we serve.

These core values help the practice create a mission statement, which is designed to reflect core values in action. It describes what we want to be and how we plan on achieving that.

We are veterinary professionals dedicated to providing compassionate, quality pet care in a manner that reflects our responsibility to those that visit our practice and to each other. We will be financially responsible with our resources, innovative in our approach to veterinary medicine, and caring in all that we do.

Our core values also help us create our vision statement, which is a public-facing statement that describes the ideal role of the practice in the community:

Our vision is to have an acclaimed veterinary practice, known for its quality medical care, advanced services, and caring attitude. We want to be the veterinary practice of choice for our region, the place to which people bring their pets with confidence and about which they tell their friends.

Although these may appear to be words on a page, we endeavor to live them as we work day to day. We cannot succeed at our mission unless, acting as responsible individuals, we form a strong team and coordinate our efforts toward our goal. This manual will help you understand your responsibilities and the requirements of your position, but never lose sight of the fact that you are part of a team effort. You will need to rely on others, and they will be relying on you every day.

YOUR ROLE ON OUR TEAM

At its most basic, our veterinary practice helps owners with their pets' health care needs. We provide a variety of medical and surgical care, appropriate products, services, and education to help pets live happy, healthy lives. We see many clients and

1

pets each day, and each of them has unique needs. As you grow to understand the value and extent of the human–animal bond, you will begin to understand the big picture of what you do each day. Because it would be impossible for one person to adequately hold all these responsibilities, we rely on a team approach. Your position in our practice is similar to a position on a sports team. The team will do well when all the individuals are performing at their best.

> *"It is rewarding to me to know that I have contributed to a patient's care. I'm proud to work among highly trained doctors and technicians that bring an intensity and integrity to their craft. I'm moved by their empathy and care and thrilled when I see a happy pet greet his owner at discharge. It's challenging but in the back of my mind is the thought that helping the client helps the pet and there is no other job that could bring me as much satisfaction as this."*
>
> —SUSAN SMITH, NORTHEAST VETERINARY REFERRAL HOSPITAL

Your Primary Responsibility

Although we will break your job down into many tasks that you need to learn, we want you to understand your primary responsibility: *Use all of your talents to create a positive environment in which the team is able to meet the needs and expectations of our clients, their pets, and our practice.*

In essence, by hiring you for this position, we are purchasing your time to help us meet this goal. We understand that ultimately this will mean a balancing act among your personal needs, the team's needs, and your job description. At times, this balancing act may require special changes, but ultimately the bargain and expectation are that you will trade your time and be paid for helping us create a great experience for our clients and their pets. That expectation is congruent with our core values and mission and vision statements, and will help you build a rewarding professional career at our practice.

Your Job Description

The individuals at our practice work as a team, and, just like a sports team, each has a position to which he or she has been assigned. You have accepted the position of CSR, and in our practice a CSR is responsible for certain tasks. The team's success will depend on your ability to learn and accomplish these tasks in a manner that allows you to live up to your primary responsibility as described previously. A basic sample of a CSR job description is given in Figure 1.1.

FIGURE 1.1 CSR Job Description

CSR Job Description

Primary Responsibility
- Interact with clients and other team members to create high-quality pet health care and great client service.

Main Job Tasks and Responsibilities
- Provide caring, compassionate service to clients by telephone or face-to-face.
- Use the veterinary software to appropriately enter client data and schedule appointments.
- Accurately process client payments.
- Resolve minor client complaints or refer the problem to a supervisor.
- Help create accurate, timely medical records.
- Create a warm, friendly, and welcoming environment.
- Communicate clearly with clients, team, and other members of the veterinary community.

Education and Experience
- High school diploma, general education degree, or equivalent
- Knowledge of client service principles and practices
- Computer skills, including Word and Excel functions

Key Competencies
- Communication skills
- Compassionate and caring attitude
- Attention to detail and accuracy
- Strong client service orientation
- Ability to react with grace under stressful conditions

Your Training Schedule

As you can see, there is a great deal involved in your job description, and to accomplish these lofty goals, you will need to learn many tasks and perform them with speed, accuracy, and grace. In order to help you absorb this amount of information, we want you to learn your tasks in stages, which we represent as training levels. Some of the tasks you will learn are presented in the following sample training schedule.

FIGURE 1.2 Client Service Task Training Timeline

Your First Week

This week will be your general orientation to our practice. You will need to:

- Know the important information about the practice: its name, location (address and local landmarks), the owners and associate veterinarians, and general services.
- Know the facility's layout and location of service areas.
- Understand our general safety procedures, including location of all the safety equipment and the evacuation protocol.
- Be familiar with our medical record system, including how we store client and patient data and where information is entered.
- Be familiar with the computer system and associated software.
- Be familiar with our phone system and related policies, including identification of various lines, placing callers on hold, and taking messages.
- Be familiar with the clinic environment, including proper cleanliness, location of cleaning products, and how the client service area should be maintained.

Your First Month

In addition to the tasks listed above, by the end of your first month, you should:

- Be familiar with the practice information and able to share it clearly and concisely with clients, including offering directions from several directions.
- Know how to accurately schedule clients for all types of appointments.
- Know how to invoice clients for services and properly collect payments.
- Communicate the value of the veterinary services performed at our practice at all times during phone conversations or face-to-face encounters.
- Understand the computer software tasks directly associated with the CSR position, including how we enter client notes, how we make financial corrections in the computer or paper record, how we review the patient's medical history, and where the vaccination history is located.
- Provide clients with basic discharge information and general information on the basic veterinary procedures we offer.

Your Third Month

In addition to the tasks listed above, by the end of the third month, you should:

- Know all the practice's major policies and procedures as they relate to your job position, including financial policies, client service policies, and facility policies.
- Know the format and layout of the patient's medical record.
- Answer client questions about the most often offered medical services and products and know why they are important and their value to the client and pet.
- Handle with grace a challenging client situation, including listening to concerns, explaining our policies, and, when necessary, deferring their concerns to the proper supervisor.
- Recognize patient medical emergencies and respond appropriately.
- Accurately provide financial information to clients, including processing invoices, completing transactions, and finalizing end-of-day financial procedures.

Other Responsibilities

Please remember that in accordance with your primary responsibility to "use all of your talents to create a positive environment in which the team is able to meet the needs and expectations of our clients, their pets, and our practice" and perform the job descriptive tasks listed, you will be asked to learn additional information about our practice and how it works. These various learning experiences will help you to understand the value you bring to the lives of our clients and their pets and enrich your professional life. They might include attending local career fairs to speak about the veterinary practice, participating in a local dog walkathon, helping to plan the holiday party, or cross-training to help with other job duties at the practice.

A Final Thought

You may be feeling overwhelmed with all this information. Take a breath; we want you to be successful. The greater your contribution to our practice, the better equipped our practice will be to complete our mission and achieve our vision.

In your endeavor to learn and become a vital member of our team, your top priorities for each day should be as follows:

- **Come to the practice ready to learn.** Arrive on time, alert, and appropriately dressed.
- **Be pleasant.** Learning is stressful, and undoubtedly there will be times you feel overwhelmed, but always try to wear a smile.
- **Give your best effort.** Be attentive and try to understand and retain the items that you are being taught. If something doesn't make sense, ask your trainer to review the process with you again.
- **Be a part of the team.** One of the most stressful parts of a new job is assimilating into the group. Look for ways to be friendly, perhaps by eating lunch with the group or saying hello and introducing yourself to new faces.
- **Enjoy your new position.** Congratulate yourself on attaining this position. You have joined a great group of people in a great profession who work hard to make life better for the people and pets they serve. Come join us in our efforts to have an impact on the lives of our clients, our patients, and our world.

HOW YOU WILL BE EVALUATED

We need you to be successful in learning your job tasks and understanding your job responsibilities as soon as possible. In order to monitor your learning, we will evaluate your progress.

At the end of your first week, you will meet with your supervisor and another CSR or team member. During this meeting, we will ask for feedback from you and provide you with feedback on your progress. We will review your job description and your learning schedule, noting which tasks you have mastered and on which you are still progressing. We will set goals for our next evaluation.

At the end of one month, we will meet again and review your training schedule, your progress, and your team contributions. You should have accomplished all the tasks addressed in the one-month phase training program. If, at any time, what you are being asked to do is unclear, ask your supervisor to explain.

At the end of three months, you will be tested on tasks for which you should have gained competency and your overall progress will be evaluated. You may be asked to take a competency test or to perform particular tasks while being observed by your supervisor. You will most likely be evaluated by two' or three individuals with whom you work frequently.

Additional reviews will take place as necessary. Yearly evaluations are standard at our practice; however, the management team is always reviewing the team's performance and may give you feedback at any time. Please remember that we have an open-door policy that allows you to approach your supervisor when you have questions or concerns about your work.

This standard procedure does not modify the disciplinary procedures or the employment-at-will policy outlined in your employee handbook.

> *Being a CSR is rewarding, pleasing, and fulfilling. I greet the client and guide them through their appointment. The level of support I offer sets the tone for the remainder of their visit and results in better health care, a happy client, and a successful outcome. Bonding with clients is the highlight of any CSR's day."*
>
> —VANESSA LESPERANCE, VALLEY CENTRAL VETERINARY REFERRAL CENTER

We hope that this brief introduction along with your orientation will help you feel acclimated to your new professional surroundings. Veterinary medicine is a challenging field full of rewarding experiences. We want you to feel welcome and excited about your new position. We work as a team and will be expecting you to grow more and more capable in your job-related tasks and in your overall value as a member of our team. Welcome aboard.

CHAPTER TWO

Information Every Team Member Should Know

Individuals in any profession eventually become skilled at certain tasks, develop particular knowledge, and become able to provide specific services. In the process, they develop bodies of information, vocabulary, guidelines, and protocols. As a new CSR, you will need to assimilate basic information about the veterinary profession that will help you build a strong foundation for your growth in our practice.

A BRIEF HISTORY OF VETERINARY MEDICINE

In a nutshell, the profession of veterinary medicine can be described as animal health care. It encompasses medical, surgical, diagnostic, preventive, and therapeutic practices that may be directed toward helping animals that are wild, domesticated (livestock and working animals), or companion animals. Veterinary professionals also address concerns as they arise from our relationship with animals and play a key role in food safety and public health. According to the American Veterinary Historical Society, "The profession has boosted static economies, assured war victories, provided safe meat and dairy products, helped build thriving livestock industries, and has been instrumental in the development of human health measures."[3]

Many years ago, when most Americans lived on farms, a veterinarian's primary focus was on livestock and horse care. Keeping the working and the food animals healthy, the sole practitioner traveled through rural areas. It meant long hours and hard physical work. As little as fifty years ago, it was rare for veterinarians to work exclusively with companion animals, and as little as thirty years ago, it was rare that you would find a female veterinarian. As you can see from the practice you are joining, the veterinary profession has changed greatly.

Today's typical veterinary practice may focus on large (e.g., cows, sheep), equine (horses), exotic (e.g., birds, reptiles, fish), or companion (cats, dogs, and small pocket pets) animals or combine several of these areas within one practice. There may be one, two, or many veterinarians accompanied by a team of support staff. The veterinarians themselves may address general practice or become specialized in one of twenty veterinary specialties, including anesthesiology, behavior, dermatology, emergency and critical care, internal medicine, cardiology, oncology, ophthalmology, neurology, radiology, and surgery, recognized by the American Veterinary Medical Association (AVMA).

THE HUMAN–ANIMAL BOND

Although you may never have heard the term, if you're a pet lover, you already have some understanding of the human–animal bond. Scientifically described, it is the interchange between people and animals that creates a dynamic and mutually beneficial relationship. It includes physical, emotional, and psychological components[4] and is a powerful contributor to the daily routine of a veterinary practice. More metaphysically, it is the connection between people and their pets.

The human–animal bond will influence your clients, their pets, and your team on a daily basis. When you see the individual who struggles emotionally to let go and leave her pet at our facility for the day, you are seeing the human–animal bond; when your team members cry during a euthanasia, you are seeing an aspect of the human–animal bond; and when a client struggles to find the finances to pay for her pet's surgical procedure, you are witnessing a component of the human–animal bond. Don't ever forget that you cannot know how the bond is affecting another individual. A key component of being a good veterinary client service professional is understanding that the bond between your client and her pet may involve myriad emotional and psychological components. Be respectful of its power to move people to do great or distressing things.

VETERINARY TERMINOLOGY

Every profession creates a vocabulary that is specific to its daily routines. These words may be unfamiliar to those who do not regularly encounter them and may seem daunting and difficult. The veterinary profession is no different. As you spend time with those who work in veterinary medicine, you will learn many terms and their pronunciation. As you begin, do your best to learn what they mean and the proper way to say each of these terms. Below is a beginning vocabulary list for you to study, starting with job titles.

Veterinary Job Titles

Specific job titles refer to the skills and responsibilities of the individuals who carry them. Familiarity with this information will help guide you through each day as you interact with your team members and the veterinary profession at large. The following is a basic list of job titles in the veterinary profession:

- **Veterinarian (pronounced vet-er-uh-nair-ee-uhn.**[5] A veterinarian is a person qualified and authorized to practice veterinary medicine. A veterinarian has attended undergraduate studies before entering veterinary school and will complete approximately four years of advanced study in veterinary medicine. There are more than twenty-five accredited colleges of veterinary medicine in the United States and additional colleges in Canada and other countries. Veterinarians may work in a variety of settings, including private or public practice, research, teaching, military service, and public health. In order to practice veterinary medicine, individuals must be licensed by the state in which they work. They will be required to attend continuing education courses to stay current with medical advancements and are subject to regulation by the state under a Veterinary Practice Act.

- **Specialist.** As defined by the AVMA in their Model Practice Act, a "veterinary specialist" is a veterinarian who has been awarded and maintains certification from an AVMA-recognized veterinary specialty organization."[6] These veterinarians have specialized in a particular aspect of veterinary medicine and have chosen to continue their education through an internship or residency in one of the twenty veterinary specialties recognized by the AVMA. You may have veterinary specialists in anesthesiology, behavior, dermatology, emergency and critical care, internal medicine, cardiology, oncology, ophthalmology, neurology, radiology, or surgery as part of your veterinary community. These individuals work alongside the general practitioner to augment care for pets by providing specialty services much as in human medicine. For more information on veterinary specialists, refer to the AVMA website (www.avma.org).

- **Veterinary Technician.** A veterinary technician has been trained in the basic principles of animal life processes, knows how to care for and handle animals, and performs laboratory and clinical procedures under the supervision of a veterinarian. By law, veterinary technicians are not allowed to diagnose, prescribe, perform surgery, or engage in any activity prohibited by a state's practice act. It is important to note here that states may designate as veterinary technicians those who have met specific criteria. In general, those who have completed two to four years of education at an approved school and have passed the Veterinary Technician National Exam may be licensed by their state and be called Certified (CVT), Registered (RVT), or Licensed (LVT) Veterinary Technicians. Some practices designate all individuals supporting the veterinarian by providing direct animal care as veterinary technicians. Others reserve the title for those individuals who have passed their state's licensing requirements and prefer to call nonlicensed individuals by the title veterinary assistant.

- **Veterinary Technician Specialist.** Specialty training in the field of veterinary technology is available for the following areas of veterinary medicine: dental technology, anesthesia, surgery, internal medicine, emergency and critical care, clinical practice, nutrition, behavior, zoological medicine, clinical pathology, and equine veterinary nursing. These individuals are licensed veterinary technicians who have extended their education to include specialized training, testing, and certification. The National Association of Veterinary Technicians in America lists the requirements for veterinary technician specialists and updates their website with new specialties as they are created.

- **Veterinary Assistant.** Veterinary assistants are individuals working within the practice to support the veterinarian and veterinary technician. Typically they work directly with animals and in some practices may be called kennel assistants. Their job responsibilities may differ greatly among practices.

- **CSR.** Sometimes also called a receptionist, the client service personnel at a veterinary practice are the client's first and last impression of the entire team. They may greet, answer questions from, attend to, and collect payment from the client. They facilitate communication throughout the practice and beyond, extending their influence to the local veterinary community and general population of their town or city.

- **Practice Manager or Hospital Administrator.** Every great team needs a leader, and the practice manager or the hospital administrator is the leader for the practice's organizational team. These individuals may have additional managers working alongside them to provide management of functions such as human resources, practice operations, budget and inventory management, and accounting.

Veterinary Medical Terminology

The following is a short list of veterinary-specific terms to get you started. You will find other terms defined throughout this manual. You will also need to become familiar with veterinary abbreviations. At the back of this book is a list of abbreviations you may encounter in the medical records or notes of our practice. It includes abbreviations for the various species of pets, pharmacology instructions, common diagnostics, and many of the procedures you may see happening within our practice.

- **Canine.** Canine is the species name for dogs. Your software will list dogs as Canine or (K9).
- **Feline.** Feline is the species name for cats. Your software will list cats as Feline or (FE).
- **DSH.** Many breed names will be abbreviated for daily use. DSH stands for domestic shorthair. This would indicate a mixed-breed cat with short hair. It may be of one or many colors.
- **Spay.** Spay is the common term for a female that has been sterilized through ovario-hysterectomy (removal of the ovaries and uterus).
- **Neuter.** Neuter is the common term for males that have been sterilized by castration.
- **Heartworm.** Heartworm is a parasitic disease that is spread by mosquitoes and can cause life-threatening illness.
- **CBC.** CBC is an abbreviation for complete blood count. This is a diagnostic blood test commonly performed in veterinary medicine.

You will encounter may more terms during your time with us. Feel free to ask a veterinarian or teammate to explain any term you do not understand or look it up in a veterinary dictionary.

PREVENTIVE CARE

Just as in human medicine, veterinarians recommend regular checkups and preventive care for pets. Many of the clients you encounter will be looking for these services. Your ability to meet their immediate needs will be enhanced by your greater knowledge of these common medical situations. What follows is a general guide to some of the situations you may encounter.

Preventive Health Visits

Our pets cannot speak to us to let us know where they hurt, what doesn't feel good, or what they need. For this reason, veterinarians recommend regular wellness and preventive health visits, including comprehensive physical examinations. During the examination, the veterinarian will collect environmental (e.g., What does she eat? Does she go outdoors?) and medical (e.g., When were her last vaccinations? How are her stools?) histories from the owner. The pet's vital parameters will be checked and recorded, including temperature, weight, heart rate, and pulse. The veterinarian will check the pet's body systems and input the results of the examination in the pet's medical record. As pets progress through their life, they require different types of medical monitoring. Just as in humans, at a certain age certain diagnostic tests are recommended. Our practice follows "life-stage" comprehensive examination recommendations. You should become familiar with these so you can explain them to clients, but at this point in your training, you only need to understand that the veterinarian may recommend different diagnostic testing or procedures depending on the age of the pet.

Some life-stage recommendations are part of our puppy and kitten protocols, such as a schedule for vaccinations, nutrition advice, and routine tests like fecal examinations. Additionally, dogs and cats older than six years of age are very likely middle-aged. Typically, discussions regarding nutrition and oral care will be prudent, as well as the routine vaccination and diagnostic testing schedule.

The Importance of Vaccinations

Pets' bodies may be challenged by diseases they encounter in their environment, and without previous inoculations against such diseases, sickness and even death may occur. Our practice wants clients to bring their pets in for examination and vaccination on a regular basis depending on the pet's stage of life. Young puppies and kittens are usually examined and vaccinated at around six, nine, and twelve weeks of age. Puppies usually get one additional examination at sixteen weeks of age. The vaccinations the pet receives will be determined by the veterinarian depending on the environment in which the pet lives, its exposure to disease, and its general health. After those visits, veterinarians generally want to examine a pet twice a year and may or may not be updating vaccinations at any particular visit.

Other Components of Preventive Care

In addition to a thorough physical examination and the necessary vaccinations, the veterinarian may want to perform the following procedures and tests:

- **Fecal examination.** Pets get parasites in their intestinal tract that cause disease, decrease nutrition, and may pass between pets and people (zoonosis). The veterinarian may provide an anthelminic to treat intestinal disease.
- **External parasite examination.** In addition to internal parasites, pets get external parasites. Fleas and ticks can be very problematic depending on the pet's environ-

2

ment. Over-the-counter flea and tick preventives are often incorrectly used by the client and can result in harm to the pet or possibly death. Our practice has particular medications we recommend for our clients. Become familiar with these products and their correct application and learn how to speak intelligently about their value.

- **Nail trim, anal gland expression, and ear cleaning.** Many pets need their nails trimmed, glands expressed, or ears cleaned on a regular basis, and sometimes they don't like the process. It may be easiest for your client to bring the pet to you for these frequent procedures. Many practices will schedule these minor procedures with a technician who is qualified to work under the direction of the veterinarian.

- **Heartworm testing.** Dogs and cats are susceptible to heartworm. This is a parasite that infects the pet through the bite of an infected mosquito. There are tests to determine whether a pet has been infected by heartworm and preventive medications that can help to protect the pet. These will be components of a wellness and preventive health program for dogs and cats.

- **Dental examination.** Just as oral care is important to humans, it is important for pets as well. Our veterinarians complete oral examinations as a component of almost every physical examination. The veterinarian will look at the teeth, the gums, and the oral cavity in general. Dental radiographs may be taken.

- **Nutrition evaluation.** Good nutrition is important for normal development and good health. A pet's nutritional requirements vary at every life stage and by lifestyle. Our veterinarians review the nutritional needs of pets and make specific recommendations to owners.

- **Microchip implantation.** No matter how hard we work to prevent it, pets get lost. Microchips implanted under the skin of the pet are the best source of permanent identification. They can be placed with minor discomfort during routine examinations.

- **Other diagnostic testing.** The veterinarian may want to include basic blood or urine tests or radiographic testing as part of the practice's pet wellness and preventive health program.

Client Education

A vital component of wellness and preventive care is client education materials. These include handouts, videos, brochures, and instructions that help the client understand the imperative need for continued pet health care. As a CSR for our practice, you should become familiar with the various educational materials available for your use. Read these and familiarize yourself with the information so you may easily share it with clients.

THERAPEUTIC CARE

Despite a client's best efforts, pets get ill or injured and need medical attention. When pet owners encounter these situations, they need your help. Most likely, they have little or no understanding of what is happening to their friend and their emotions will be aroused to one extent or another. As a CSR, your attentiveness, demeanor, and helpful attitude will make all the difference in the situation. As you would suppose, sick pets need to be examined expeditiously. Scheduling a sick-patient visit is covered later, but now let's talk about what you might encounter as part of a therapeutic pet visit.

Typically, sick and injured pets need more extensive care than pets brought to the practice for wellness and preventive care. They may need to be hospitalized if your practice offers this service, or transferred to another facility for continued care.

Common Illnesses or Conditions

Some ailments and procedures are common in veterinary medicine. Although you should never attempt to diagnose what is occurring with the pet's health, it can be very helpful to understand these common situations:

- **Anal sacs.** Animals have glands on either side of their rectum that may become impacted or infected, causing pain. Typical symptoms include the pet scooting on its bottom and licking at its anal area.
- **Ear problems.** A pet's ears get dirty, and the buildup of debris may cause infection and pain. The pet may shake its head or rub its head on the floor or ground. The debris may be brown in color, of a waxy consistency, and smelly. Sometimes, especially in cats, the brown debris may be ear mites (small mites that infect the ears of pets). Hematomas may develop on the ears of pets. Typically caused by trauma to the ear flap, an ear hematoma is a buildup of blood between the layers of cartilage in the pet's ear. It looks as if the ear has blown up like a balloon.
- **Oral or dental conditions.** Pets need dental care just as humans do. They have bad breath, get cavities, break teeth, and may need more significant dental care like extractions, root canals, or caps. There are veterinary specialists who work entirely with a pet's dental problems; however, most veterinary practices perform routine dental cleaning and minor dental procedures such as extractions.
- **Internal and external parasites.**
    - **Internal.** Several types of internal parasites can affect pets, and some are transferable to humans. Roundworms, hookworms, whipworms, and tapeworms are internal parasites.

- **External.** Fleas and ticks infect both cats and dogs. Preventives are available for use depending on the size and species of the pet.
- **Vomiting and diarrhea.** Pets may experience vomiting and diarrhea for a variety of reasons, including everything from a mild upset to a life-threatening contagious disease. Read and become familiar with information on parvovirus, pancreatitis, and other common diseases that exhibit these symptoms. When you are speaking with clients about their pet's vomiting and diarrhea, be sure you ask questions that may help the doctor determine their source. Asking the patient's age; whether she is current with her vaccinations; has eaten any new foods or other odd items, including foreign objects such as bones and toys; has been exposed to other sick pets; etc., will provide valuable information for the doctors.

Common Diagnostic Procedures

Just as your physician will request blood work or Xrays when determining your state of health, veterinarians do the same for the pets they see. Diagnostics are the various forms of testing that help the doctor determine what's happening in the pet's body to create the symptoms that are manifested. Following are some of the diagnostic tests in veterinary medicine. They are comparable to human diagnostic testing and take many forms:

- **Blood analysis.** Many veterinary medical facilities have laboratory equipment capable of blood and urine analysis. Others may choose to send their blood and urine tests to laboratories outside the practice. Either way, diagnostic blood tests will help the doctor determine the underlying cause of the pet's symptoms. In-house laboratory capabilities might include the following:
  - **CBC.** This is a test that reveals the number and types of blood cells in a sample.
  - **Blood chemistry.** This blood diagnostic test is run on the fluid in the blood sample. Its results indicate liver and kidney organ function.
  - **Urinalysis.** Examining the pet's urine will give the veterinarian information about urinary tract disease and kidney disease as well as contribute information about the function of other organs.
  - **Thyroid testing.** Many veterinary hospitals can test a pet's blood for the presence of thyroid disease.
  - **Blood gases.** These can be analyzed to determine the pet's pulmonary function.
  - **Radiographs.** Many veterinary practices use digital radiography; however, conventional film radiology is still used as well. Radiographs help veterinarians diagnose skeletal injuries or abnormalities, the presence of tumors, ingestion of foreign bodies, heart enlargement, bladder stones, etc. Digital radiology uses computer imaging. Conventional film radiology uses film that is developed through a processor.

- **Ultrasonography.** Ultrasonography helps the veterinarian diagnose internal conditions that may not be seen on radiographs. Some practices have their own veterinarian interpret the ultrasound results, and others send the images to a specialist who provides the interpretation in electronic format.
- **Electrocardiography and other monitoring capabilities.** Various monitors are available in the veterinary profession to help the doctor diagnose disease. Monitors may include a visual or audio display of such vital parameters as heart rate, blood pressure, pulse, and Spo_2 (oxygen saturation as measured by pulse oximetry), and may be used during surgical procedures or to monitor hospitalized patients.

Our practice has many of these capabilities on the premises.

HOSPITALIZATION

Many practices hospitalize patients overnight. Patients may be housed in specific wards or in the general population. They may be medicated or have diagnostic testing and treatments performed by the veterinary staff over the course of their hospitalization. Clients will want to know about changes in their pet's condition, thus necessitating continual client communication with you and the veterinary staff.

During hospitalization at our practice, the following safety procedures are followed:

- All patients are monitored by technicians 24/7.
- There is a veterinarian on the premises 24/7.
- Monitoring machines such as electrocardiography and Spo_2 monitors are available 24/7.
- All procedures and medications are documented in the medical record and on treatment sheets (paper or electronic) that are checked continually by the nursing team.
- Clients may check on a pet's condition at any time and will receive regular follow-up calls by the veterinarian or another team member.

SURGICAL PROCEDURES

Surgical procedures are performed on pets in much the same way as in human hospitals. Pets are given anesthesia and pain medications and are monitored by experienced technical team members. Many of your clients will be nervous about leaving their pet for surgery, afraid that something dire will occur. Although all surgery has an element of danger, veterinarians will thoroughly discuss the benefits of each procedure with the pet's owner. You should become familiar with the types of surgery performed at our practice and the procedures our team performs to do our best to ensure that each patient's surgical experience is as uneventful as possible. Routine surgical procedures include the following:

- **Castration.** Surgical removal of the testicles resulting in sterility for male cats and dogs is called castration.
- **Spaying.** Surgical removal of the ovaries resulting in sterility for female cats and dogs is called ovariohysterectomy or spaying.
- **Declawing.** Some practices declaw cats by surgically removing their claws.

During every surgical procedure, our practice follows the guidelines outlined below to ensure patient safety:

- We follow industry-accepted guidelines for patient safety.
- We perform presurgical blood analysis on all surgical patients.
- We use patient-warming devices for anesthetic procedures.
- We perform continual patient monitoring by electrocardiography, end-tidal CO_2 (the level of CO_2 released at the end of expiration), Spo_2 monitors, blood pressure monitors, and individually assigned technicians.
- We have designated recovery room technical team members who monitor patients.

WHAT CONSTITUTES AN EMERGENCY

Every new CSR worries that she won't be able to recognize an emergency when it happens. We all know that when a pet is bleeding profusely, having trouble breathing, is unconscious or having seizures, or is unable to stand up, the pet needs immediate care, but what about those more subtle things that could be life-threatening? Chapters 4 and 5 include in-depth information on how to help clients who call or come in with potential emergencies, but provided here are examples of common situations to watch for:

- **Bloat.** Bloat is a condition involving the gastrointestinal system. It typically affects larger dogs and is typically indicated by distension of the dog's abdomen, but the pet can present with many different symptoms. It is life-threatening unless immediate action is taken by the veterinary team.
- **Urinary blockage.** When the urethra of the pet is obstructed (typically caused by grit or stones that have formed in the urinary tract), a urinary blockage occurs. This condition is fairly frequent among the male cat population. Unless treated promptly, the pet could die.

- **Heatstroke.** Pets left in the sun too long, walked too vigorously on a hot day, or left in the car may experience a life-threatening increase in body temperature. This can be evidenced by a loud pant and a frantic expression or attitude. If untreated, a significant increase in temperature will result in a coma and death.
- **Trauma.** Perhaps the pet has been hit by car, fallen from a height, been in a fight, or been stepped or fallen on. It is always recommended that trauma patients be seen. These patients can have hidden injuries, such as internal hemorrhage, pneumothorax, pulmonary contusions, or traumatic brain injury, that can get worse over the first twenty-four to forty-eight hours.

There are many more potentially life-threatening illnesses you may encounter. The doctors and medical team will help you determine which conditions require immediate medical action.

Be aware that *anything* may be an emergency to a client who is experiencing abnormal behavior of her pet. Clients panic with pets just as parents panic with children. Your position, as a CSR, is to *remain calm* and seek medical personnel to reassure the client. You can be a calming influence to the client. No matter whether the situation is an emergency you can identify from the previous list or just a client in distress, call for medical backup and let the trained personnel decide. This lets the client know that you are immediately helping her and that the pet will be assessed by a member of the medical team.

———

As you can see, there is much for you to learn as you begin your career associated with the veterinary profession. In this chapter, we have provided you with an overview of the job titles and primary topics that will occupy your daily routine at the practice. Become as familiar as you can with these topics. They will provide a good foundation for your future with us.

How Would You Define *Client Service?*

Typically veterinary hospitals have used the term *client* for the patrons who visit their practice. The definition of *client* denotes a somewhat dependent relationship in which the service provider has a professional responsibility to the patron. *Merriam-Webster's Collegiate Dictionary* defines *client* in this way: "A person who engages the professional advice or services of another."[7] The implication is that the professional knows something the client doesn't and provides services to meets the client's needs.

A *customer*, on the other hand, is defined by the same source as "one that purchases a commodity or service." It implies that there is less responsibility to the purchaser. Thus, the attorney has clients, the doctor has clients, and the retail store and gas station have customers.

This distinction is important for you to remember as you go about your daily duties. For the hospital mission to be successful, each member of the veterinary team needs to treat the patron as a client. You have a professional responsibility to meet the patron's needs as they fall within the bounds of the practice's mission and your position at the practice. Striving to meet the client's expectations is the best definition of client service.

ALL BUSINESS IS SHOW BUSINESS

All business is show business. We live in an entertainment culture where every business is expected to connect with our personal needs. We expect the business to provide not just the service we came for but all the extras as well. As consumers, we used to accept some of the undesirable side stuff as a necessary evil to get the service we were seeking. Now, we want to get something out of every interaction, and we intend to tell others about whether our experience was good or bad. We no longer get our car fixed at the greasy garage. We want a lounge in which to sit, with coffee and TV. An individual used to come to a veterinary hospital strictly for veterinary care. They would not care whether the veterinarian's office smelled like chemicals and medications and dogs and cats. But today, we have refined the buying–purchasing scenario into the total experience. In 2002, when the book *All Business Is Show Business*[8] was published, the Retail Marketing Institute released a study saying that more than 70 percent of customers would go somewhere else to make a purchase if it was more "entertaining" to do business elsewhere.

In today's consumer culture, clients have become even more accustomed to a total-experience veterinary visit. This puts a lot of pressure on CSRs. Clients will judge our veterinary practice as much on the waiting room as they do on the medicine, as much on the bedside manner of the veterinarian as on his knowledge. Your abilities as a CSR directly affect the profitability of our practice, and you are always on stage.

CLIENT EMOTIONS AND EXPECTATIONS

Your clients are people just like you. As they arrive at your front door, they are bringing with them not only their pet but also everything that has happened to them before their visit to our practice. They may be hurried or relaxed, nervous or expectant. They may be feeling ill, or they may have had everything go their way that day and be feeling on top of the world.

They may also have already imagined what will happen during their visit to our practice and have expectations. Their expectations may be founded on other experiences they have had in veterinary offices, a friend's recollection of their experience at our practice, an advertisement they have seen, or the conversation they had with one of our team. These expectations may be positive, so they are pleasantly excited about their visit; neutral, with a wait-and-see attitude; or negative, so they come in the door with a chip on their shoulder. Whatever their experience, they walk over to you carrying some expectation.

This is the greatest client service dilemma: Everyone has different life experiences and develops different expectations. No two people coming through our doors are going to share the same set of life circumstances, be in the same mood, or have the same expectations. How, then, are you ever to meet their expectations and respond to their needs? The best method is to develop an understanding of some of the factors that influence our clients and use this understanding to provide great customer service at all times. The remainder of this chapter attempts to show you how.

THE PSYCHOLOGY OF MONEY

No matter how you put it, veterinary care costs money. And just all our clients comes through our door with expectations, they all carry emotions about money. Some of these emotions may go way back in their history, so you will not be able to evaluate or understand them. You just have to know how to recognize some of the pitfalls those emotions may bring to your tasks as a CSR.

Money is an objective thing. Everyone has a certain amount. You can count it. Emotions belong to the individual and are very subjective. We cannot fathom another's deepest emotions. So when a client comes to the front desk to pay for services, you can see his money but you cannot know how the transaction is affecting him psychologically. Economists argue that money acts as a tool for us to achieve our goals, but some psychologists go further to say that money acts as a drug. It can change how we feel. Recent studies suggest that people who are sad seek change and spend their money more thoughtlessly, people who are disgusted want to get rid of everything, and people who are anxious want to reduce the anxiety and may soothe themselves with low-risk buying.[9] So, too, others hang on to money and hoard or save beyond normal or healthy limits. We have probably all experienced how our emotions affect what we spend.

Our practice has SOPs for payment policies used within the practice. It will be helpful, as you adhere to those policies, to understand that "when clients vent frustration, it is usually more about them than it is about you."[10]

Clients may react negatively because of any of the following factors:

- **Their underlying insecurities about money.** Your clients may react negatively to paying you what they owe, even though they understood and agreed to the services. They may be crabby about the bill, make comments about the high cost of care, and reluctantly hand over their payment. Many times these statements do not reflect their true feelings about the care their pet received but rather on how hard it is for them to part with money.
- **Their feelings of inadequacy, embarrassment, or guilt.** When unable to pay for the *best* care for their pet, clients may strike out at you, accusing you of lack of compassion because you won't perform free services.

In these situations it is best to acknowledge what the client is feeling by saying something like "I can see that you are surprised by the total on your invoice." And offer to help them better understand the charges on the invoice: "We want you to be satisfied with the care we give to Fluffy. Do you have questions about today's visit that I might help you with?" Or "I know that you care for Fluffy and that this situation was unplanned. Finances are always a difficult part of my job. I love animals and feel sad when we can't help them for free. Unfortunately, we both have to work within financial constraints, but let's see if we can put our heads together to give Fluffy the best that we can."[11] For more tips, refer to "Talking to Clients About Payment" in Chapter 8.

THE BASICS OF GREAT CLIENT SERVICE

All great client service has its foundation in some basic elements and actions that create a connection between individuals. Although some personality characteristics predispose individuals to a warm, friendly nature, all the techniques that improve client service outcomes can be learned by those with a true desire to improve their interpersonal communication abilities. Becoming competent in these techniques will help you progress at our practice and in your professional career.

First Impressions Matter

First impressions can make or break your relationship with an individual. The same is true for businesses. Our first impression will be a lasting impression. A client gets blasted with sensory data when he walks in our door. The client's first environmental impression of our practice needs to be a good one. Take a moment and walk in the door of the practice. What do you notice? Is the room friendly-looking, is there an odor, are the decorations pleasing, and is the floor clean? One of your duties is to keep this area as attractive as possible. Take pride in your showroom; keep it in mint condition, and if new items are necessary, don't be afraid to make suggestions to your manager. In addition to recognizing the environmental impact of the veterinary reception area, remember that our clients evaluate your ability and professionalism by your appearance. We appreciate that you take pride in your appearance and we have created a dress code to help you understand our expectations of professional appearance (see SOP 3.1 at the end of this chapter).

Be Friendly

When someone walks in, be sure to look up and greet him as he approaches your station. Even if you are on the phone with a caller, look at the client and smile. Studies show that people react to facial features and expressions even before hearing someone speak. Babies recognize emotions in others at an early age and react accordingly. Scientists have studied brain receptors called mirror neurons. It is thought that these neurons help us to understand others and in fact can lead us to mirror others' actions and feelings.[12] They are designed to interpret the facial expressions of others and mimic them back. If you want your client to smile at you, smile at him as he comes through the door.

When you are answering the phone, the same principles apply. Your facial expression and the emotions underlying it will influence the tone of voice with which you answer the phone. Maintaining a "smiling attitude" accompanied by a smiling expression creates a pleasant, upbeat tone in your voice. Clients will hear that welcoming tone in your greeting, and the relationship will be off to a good start. Set yourself up for success on the phone by beginning with a warm pleasant greeting.

Use Clients' and Pets' Names

People like to be recognized. The theme song from the long-running sitcom *Cheers* said it all. We feel more comfortable when people call us by name.

Today, many software programs allow for pictures to be uploaded to the client's files. If this is true for your practice, avail yourself of this memory help. Look at the upcoming appointments and begin to recognize your clients. Call them and their pet by name. Speak directly to them in a clear voice with a cadence they can understand. Be careful not to speak too quickly. Hold their eye contact. Be respectful of their time and comfort level in our practice. If it is their first time, quickly explain what is going to happen: "Ms. Smith, welcome to our practice. I see that you have an appointment with Dr. Bob. He is currently with another patient. If you can have a seat in the waiting area, a technician will come out to get you shortly. If you need anything before he comes out, just let me know." This brief description puts the client at ease and tells him what to do if something doesn't feel right (see SOP 3.2 at the end of this chapter).

Be Courteous

Courteous, respectful, and polite behavior is a requirement of good client service. Although most people accept the use of common names and familiar gestures as signs of friendliness, lack of courtesy and common polite behavior is never overlooked. As the first face of our practice, always exhibit the utmost courtesy toward our clients. If you need them to do something, ask them, don't tell them. "Go sit over there" is impolite. "Would you please have a seat in the waiting area" is a courteous request. "Hold a moment" is impolite, whereas "Can you hold for a moment?" is respectful. Clients are guests in the practice, not relatives; you should treat them as a proper guest. If you are talking with a coworker when a client approaches, stop immediately and recognize the client and ask what you can do to help. Again, the same principles apply when you are talking with clients on the phone.

You may encounter someone whose native language is not English. If you have trouble understanding his needs, politely ask another team member to help you. Again, apologize and be sincere. "Let me get Jane to help us, Mr. Smith. I'm sure she will know how to solve your dilemma." Alert the other team member to the difficulty you are having without saying anything in front of the client. If you were to say, "I can't understand Mr. Smith," it might be offensive to your client. Quietly let Jane know you are having trouble understanding Mr. Smith's request.

Manage Your Time Well

Time is a limited resource in today's society. Respect our clients' time (and the practice's investment in you) by being efficient. As much as possible be ready for clients when they come into the practice. If you use hard-copy files, have patient records ready ahead of the appointment time, keep the doctor on time, and have necessary updating forms ready. Once you have greeted clients, move to expedite their visit at the practice. Refrain from personal conversations with other team members while in the reception area, especially in the presence of clients. Your focus should be on meeting clients' needs.

Be Accurate

As a CSR, you will be charged with a great deal of data collection and data entry. As service professionals in a medical field, we must reduce inaccuracies. At best, inaccuracies will frustrate clients or team members; at worst they might jeopardize a patient's health. As you can see, accuracy is important. When taking data from clients, whether in person or over the phone, focus your attention on listening to what they say. When entering data in the computer, check or repeat the information you have entered. If you take information from a client regarding the pet's health, repeat it back to the client to be sure you have understood and recorded things correctly. Focus on the task at hand, and double-check your work.

Be Knowledgeable

As you start in your client service position, you won't know much about our practice. During orientation, you were familiarized with the most pertinent aspects of our facility. This book should acquaint you with other aspects of your job and the veterinary profession. But no matter how much your trainers try to teach you as you start, there will always be more to learn. Your clients expect you to know *everything* about the practice. As you start out, don't be afraid to let them know you are new and always seek confirmation from your trainer before telling a client anything you are not 100 percent sure about. Always strive to learn more so that you can be a better asset to the practice and more helpful to your clients. Keep a notebook as a reference for more complex protocols, and review the employee handbook and client service SOPs for our practice. Ask questions and make an effort to learn as much as possible. Your position will be very rewarding as you grow to be your clients' best resource.

Be Focused

Like all areas of the practice, the client service area will have busy times and slow times. When you are busy, you will be required to juggle different tasks at once. While our culture teaches us to pride ourselves on our ability to multitask, there is a time and a place to do so. If you are working directly with a client, focus your attention on that client. Do not attempt to do two or three things at once. The client will feel disrespected, and you will be prone to make mistakes.

As a CSR, your primary concern is the clients and pets that arrive at our practice. Keep them as safe, comfortable, and relaxed as possible. During slower times, your secondary responsibilities might include keeping the area clean, keeping paperwork up-to-date, processing patient visit reminders, ordering supplies, etc. Personal business (discussion with another team member) should be stopped whenever a client is present. We all like a pleasant work environment and want to be friendly with our teammates, but clients must come first.

COMMON CHALLENGES DURING CLIENT INTERACTIONS

We previously discussed the power of the human–animal bond, the strong feelings of love and companionship that can develop between a person and a pet, and how a client's emotions and expectations may affect him during his practice experience. If the client's pet is well, he may be anxious about the doctor uncovering something unexpected; if the pet is sick, he may be even more fearful. Additional anxiety may occur if the client has an ill child or is worried about losing his job. Or the client may be happy because it is his birthday. You really don't know and cannot judge what might motivate your clients to behave in the manner they do. The important thing to remember is that although you cannot know what is happening inside them or how they will react, you can help them understand the present experience. The following sections offer situation-specific techniques to help you help your clients.

Helping Grieving Clients

Pet loss is an inevitable part of veterinary medicine. Companion animals typically have shorter life spans than their human owners, and euthanasia is an accepted practice in veterinary medicine. Both of these factors mean that you will have to work with grieving clients. At times you may be uncomfortable, and that is normal. Many people experience discomfort when facing strong emotions in the presence of others. In part, this may be due to the false belief that manifesting a grief response demonstrates personal weakness, when in fact repressing typical reactions like crying and sadness may hinder personal healing. No matter the cause, it is best that you learn to work through any discomfort you might feel.

Grieving individuals, including clients who have received bad news about their beloved pet, want and need to be supported. They want to see your acknowledgment of their plight, your respect for them and their pet, and your compassion and sincerity. You can use both verbal and nonverbal cues to convey support. Your voice tone and words can reflect warmth and empathy. Offer assistance only if needed. Ask if they would like help or would prefer to be alone. When you speak to these clients, do so clearly, honestly, and with sincerity. No matter how tempted you are to provide advice or to use clichés such as "time will heal," refrain from doing so. Grief is an individual process. It takes many forms, and for most individuals it proceeds naturally through several stages. Your clients will need to negotiate these stages in their own time and in their own manner. You cannot control their reactions, but you can offer support and help them understand the situation.

When working with grieving individuals, it is helpful to understand the following support techniques:

- **Acknowledge the fact that they are grieving.**[13] You might say, "Mr. Smith, I know you loved Fluffy and I can see that you are grieving her loss."

- **Be attentive and present with your client.** Working with a grieving client is not the time to multitask. Focus on your client's needs and avoid distractions.

- **Be an active listener.** Think about what he is saying and acknowledge him with a nod or verbal affirmation as he continues the conversation. If the conversation falters, do not be afraid of the silence. Allow clients time to process their thoughts and to reminisce if they want.

- **Share your experiences.** If you can honestly and briefly relay a similar personal experience, sharing it may help your client feel less alone in his grief. You could say, "I lost my dog, Jones, last year and understand how much this type of experience can hurt." Don't go into a lot of detail and don't monopolize the conversation. Allow the individual to talk about his loss and feelings.

- **Do not judge them by their reaction.**[14] Everyone experiences grief in a different way, and the intense feelings that accompany loss may be overwhelming to your clients. They may experience guilt, anger, fear, or despair. They might yell and curse or emotionally dissolve. The depth of their feelings may be surprising. To support them, you might say, "It is okay to feel upset; many of us who work here cry at every pet's passing. Fluffy was your friend; it is normal to feel sad at a time like this."

- **Reach out.** Not all will be brave enough to ask for things they want or need at a time of crisis. Reach out to them and ask what you can do to help. Simply asking, "How would you like me to help you during this time?" or "What can I do to support you through your loss?" may provide them with an opening to reach out to you for their needs. It is okay to be honest and let them know you are unsure of how to help.

- **Restate their answer in your own words.** Because their minds are often swimming with emotion and upset, when they answer, be sure you understand what they need. You can try saying, "Mr. Smith, if I understand correctly, you want to take Fluffy home to bury her. Am I correct?" Although this may seem uncomfortable at this time, it is better to be sure you have their wishes recorded correctly than to misunderstand and make a misstep.

- **Refrain from encouraging them to get a new pet.** Remember that people process loss on their own timeline. It may be some time before your clients are ready to replace the friend they have lost. This can be seen as an attempt to replace the lost pet and may anger or further upset your clients. If they reach a time when a new pet is welcomed into their lives, it will be when they have processed the current loss.[15]

Euthanasia is a special procedure performed in veterinary medicine to relieve a pet's suffering. It can be an intensely emotional process, and our practice endeavors to embody it with the respect due to our clients and their pets. We have developed a method of working with clients in these situations. A sample SOP for providing client care during euthanasia appointments is included at the end of this chapter (see SOP 3.3). Becoming familiar with our processes before you encounter the emotion of a euthanasia appointment will help you when working with your clients.

It is important to remember that sadness over pet death is a natural and common feeling. If you are troubled by a particular euthanasia or pet death, talk to your supervisor or manager. Compassion fatigue is real in the veterinary profession. We acknowledge that each of us is saddened by pet death and can be overcome by the feelings it brings up inside us. Talking about your feelings to your supervisor can help you clear your mind and focus on the good you do every day.

Helping Anxious or Angry Clients

A number of factors may combine to create other challenging client situations. A member of the team may have made a mistake, or the client may have perceived that a mistake was made. The client may simply have different values or communication techniques than you do and feel slighted by your tone or manner, or perhaps he felt he was made to wait too long for his visit. He may be anxious about his pet's health or something as seemingly unrelated as the cost of his mortgage. No matter the reason behind the emotion, these situations may make your day stressful and can seem overwhelming. Because several stressors may be happening at once, there is no one right way to calm everyone, but there are several behavioral tactics that can be helpful.

Even though it's hard, it's important not to take things personally. Maybe the situation reminds us of something in our past or we feel that the client is challenging our beliefs and values. If you are a very compassionate and caring individual, it is hard to listen to someone say that "all you care about is money." We may get defensive and want to protest that what he is saying isn't true. Sometimes our own emotions start to escalate.

In situations like this, remember that the client is acting out of stress; most likely his negative reaction is not related to you. Depersonalize it. Remember times when you have been stressed and reacted in a way that later looked foolish or over the top to you. If visualizations help you, think of yourself holding out a baseball catcher's mitt. Let the mitt absorb the impact of whatever the client is throwing. Just take the objective facts, the ball the client has thrown, and see what you can do to help him understand the situation. Work through the client's needs, leaving the emotion aside.

Several techniques can be used to help you remain calm and appropriately help the client:

- **Remain calm.** You can do this by quieting your breath, moving slowly through your actions, and speaking with a quiet tone and smooth delivery. Actively work to make your voice remain calm. Minimize distractions; move into a private room to speak. Focus on the other individual, but be aware of your body's reactions, breath, heart rate, and voice level (both pitch and volume). If you are getting upset and might lose control, step away from the moment. You might say, "Can you excuse me a moment? I need to check on …"

- **Don't be defensive.** There are several reasons why you might feel defensive, but the fact of the matter is that attempting to defend yourself or the practice never works. When you get defensive, the other individual will feel he needs to attack with more vigor.

- **Listen to your client; let him tell his story.** Let him play it out without interruption. Sometimes that is all he needs—just to know someone will hear him out.

- **Remain curious.** Really listen to see whether there is something you can pick up out of the conversation that will give you a cue as to why the individual is upset. Has he misunderstood something that we have said or done? Here is an example:

One practice was working with a difficult client whose pet was extremely ill. The man shouted that they were misdiagnosing his dog. He kept repeating that the doctor said the dog was only "depressed." The manager finally caught the voice inflection and the use of the word "only" before "depressed" and stopped him to explain the medical meaning of the word *depressed*, or that the pet's vital statistics were declining. That explanation clarified what the veterinarians were doing to help his pet recover and altered his demeanor during the conversation.

- **Treat clients with respect.** Even if their frustration is built out of their own performance, they should be treated respectfully. The most wonderful gift we can give to anyone, and the one they will long remember, is to be respectful when they don't deserve it. If a client loses it and yells at you for a misunderstanding, and you treat him with respect and do everything you can to satisfy him and he still leaves angry, there is a chance that he will sincerely apologize the next time you see him and thank you for your care. If you treat him disrespectfully, yelling back or acting defensively, you will probably never see him come through your doors again.

- **Ask permission to address their concerns.** Do it at that moment or let them know you will get back with them. A great tactic to manage difficult clients is the "pause." Let them vent, discuss their concerns, and take a break. It really will be good for both of you. If their concerns do not involve a simple fix, such as producing a copy of their credit card receipt, ask them for time to investigate the matter and promise to get back to them. The added advantage is that they will have time to get away from their emotions as well and will most likely calm down. *Do not forget* to respond.

- **Avoid accusatory or inflammatory words.** Examples of inflammatory words are "we never," "you always," and "your fault." Never disparage a pet. The use of words such as "aggressive" or "vicious" can inflame a pet owner.

- **Commit to help them.** This doesn't mean giving clients what they want. It just means you will help them through the situation. Many times a manager will need to call back a few days later to say that after thorough investigation of their concern, their demands cannot be met, but from the first, commit to help them better understand the situation.

- **Always follow through.** As a part of being honest to and respecting your client and being true to your word, you *must* follow through. Investigate the situation and talk to the proper individuals, but in the end *do what you said you would do*. If this is a call-back, do so within a defined time period. Try saying, "I'll need a few days to investigate all of this and talk to the right people; would it be okay if I give you a call by Monday evening?"

As you become familiar with our practice's protocols, you will be empowered to solve these dilemmas. Always follow the protocol for handling difficult clients. Refer to SOP 3.4 at the end of this chapter for a quick list of things to do when trying to help a client who is upset.

Friends of the Practice

There will undoubtedly be some clients who are "friends of the practice." They are frequent visitors and expect special treatment. You should become familiar with these clients. If you inadvertently say or do something that seems to alienate them, be forthcoming with your apology. For instance, you might say, "I'm sorry, Mr. Smith. I'm new at the practice and didn't realize that you were bringing both Fluffy and Snoopy in today."

SALES REPRESENTATIVES AND OTHER VISITORS

Along with your clients, you will be approached by or talk with sales representatives and visitors to our practice. Ask your manager if there is a specific protocol for these situations. In general, always be friendly and courteous. Ask if you can help them in order to find out who they were supposed to be seeing, whether they had an appointment, or whether they were just dropping in. Try to get their business card or full identifying information and record it accurately. If this visit is in regard to a particular pet, pull up or bring out the medical record. Next, excuse yourself to find out whether the individual was expecting this appointment and will be able to see or speak with the individual, or whether you will be required to take a message. If you will use the intercom or phone to contact your team member, step away from where the visitor is standing. Some conversations can be heard beyond the phone receiver. If you are asked to take a message, be sure to get complete information. Ask whether there are any materials the visitor would like to leave and record a best time for the visitor to be contacted by your team member.

PET VISITATION

A client whose pet is hospitalized may call or come by the practice to visit his pet. Our practice has a pet visitation policy that must be followed. Be sure you greet clients pleasantly and let them know you will notify the appropriate team members who will be able to help them. You might ask them to have a seat if it is appropriate. After notifying the medical team, follow up to be sure the clients are helped in a timely manner. Remember, everyone in the reception area is under your watch. If it appears that someone has been there a long time or is looking disturbed by the wait time, check with the appropriate team member and report back to the client about why he is still waiting and when he can expect to be called in.

Providing good client service begins with following basic client service procedures, understanding your client, and knowing yourself. The information in this chapter reviews these basic principles and will be a helpful resource for you as you learn the specific protocols for our practice. Remember that although veterinary medicine is about providing health care to pets, we will never achieve our goals without the cooperation of our clients. Reaching out to clients and helping them feel accepted and comfortable in our practice will facilitate the mission of the health care team.

❝ Being a CSR is the best job in our hospital. We need to shine everyday and promote our hospital's values and services with pride. We develop genuine caring relationships with our clients and become more than a client–receptionist partnership, we become family."

—PAULA PREIDEL, NORTHSTAR VETS

3

CHAPTER 3 SOPs

SOP 3.1: APPEARANCE STANDARDS

1. All technical staff and CSRs will be dressed in scrub uniforms that match their department's chosen color scheme. The practice will provide uniforms for team members after they have passed their introductory period. The practice will provide two uniforms for full-time team members and one uniform for part-time team members. Uniforms should be returned to the practice when team members leave employment.
2. All clothes must be appropriately laundered and pressed if necessary.
3. Name tags will be worn when you are on the floor.
4. All clothes will fit properly, including length and girth. Inappropriate views of skin will be prevented, including pants that hang too low and shirts that are too tight.
5. Jewelry should be kept to a minimum for safety reasons. No long dangly earrings. Team members involved in the surgery suite must remove inappropriate jewelry.
6. Personal hygiene will be commented on if it is not acceptable. Deodorant should be used as necessary. Hair should be combed and, if long, kept back or up out of the way. Makeup should meet professional guidelines. Fingernails should be clean and kept at an appropriate length.

If another team member notices a problem, it should be reported to the team member's direct supervisor. The supervisor should address the situation following standard management discipline guidelines. If the supervisor needs additional help, management should be consulted.

SOP 3.2: HOW TO GREET CLIENTS

Remember that you are in a "fishbowl" at the client service desk. The majority of your communication with other team members can be overheard by clients. Refrain from in-depth personal conversations when clients are present. Keep your mind on serving your clientele and completing your assigned tasks.

1. Always present a professional image. Dress modestly, professionally, and appropriately. Your supervisor will inform you of the practice's dress code. Your uniform should be clean and unwrinkled. Your hair and makeup (if applicable) should be in sync with the practice's style.

2. Make eye contact as soon as possible and smile. Turn your attention to the clients as soon as you are able. Your undivided attention will tell them you care and make them feel more comfortable.

3. Use appropriate language. Call clients by their proper title, Mr. or Ms., until they suggest a more casual relationship.

4. Greet the client and the pet. Use statements similar to "Hi, Ms. Smith, do you have Fluffy with you today?" or "Hi, Mr. Smith, how is Shadow doing?"

5. Give them appropriate direction. Verbal direction helps new clients know what is expected of them. "Ms. Smith, I have all your paperwork completed. Please have a seat in the reception area; a nurse will be with you shortly. Let me know if you need anything while you are here."

6. Be prepared to follow through with your promise. If they need water for their pet or a "cleanup" of urine or stool, take care of it or notify someone else to help them.

7. Be mindful of their wait time. If a client has been waiting more than fifteen minutes for a scheduled appointment or for information on the pet brought in for emergency treatment, seek assistance from other members of your team and get information to update the client on the reason for the wait. Most people are reasonable if they are kept informed about the circumstances surrounding the delay.

SOP 3.3: CLIENT CARE DURING EUTHANASIA

1. Whenever possible, make note of the fact that a client is coming in for a euthanasia appointment and notify the entire team. A proper respectful demeanor should be presented by all team members during euthanasia.

2. Anticipate the client's arrival. Have an open exam room or euthanasia room available for the client and pet. If at all possible, prepare a room with a blanket, more subtle lighting, tissues, and other comfort items. Let the doctor know when the client will be arriving so he can clear his schedule and the client will not be kept waiting long.

3. Greet the client with care and compassion. This may be one of the hardest things he has ever had to do and he will appreciate your understanding.

4. Consider preparing the invoice and offering to have the client take care of payment before the euthanasia so he doesn't have to stay after the procedure. Ask the client how he would like to handle the payment process.

5. If it has not been done when the appointment was scheduled, determine the client's wishes regarding the procedure. Does he want to be present or not? What will be done with the pet's body?

6. Your team should have all necessary procedural items available.

7. After the euthanasia is performed, treat the patient's body with respect and the client with care. Refer to the "Helping Grieving Clients" section of the text for more information on communicating compassion during euthanasia appointments.

SOP 3.4: HELPING CHALLENGING CLIENTS

Ask your client into an exam room or quiet area. This takes him out of the limelight, protecting other clients, lessening distractions, and removing any performance factors that might be escalating the situation.

1. Introduce yourself. Explain that you are there to help.

2. Listen to the client. Ask an open-ended question, for example, "Mr. Smith, I can see that you are upset. Would you please explain to me what has happened?" Then really listen. Be present. Do not allow distractions; keep your mind and eyes on your client. Be as empathetic as possible. You can remember times when you were the disgruntled consumer. Show the client you are listening, nod your head, and interject small verbal signposts ("Okay, and then what happened?").

3. Ask for permission to help.

4. Reiterate the facts as they have been presented by the client to be sure you understand the concerns. You must get this correct if you are to be seen as being helpful to the client.

5. Ascertain whether this is something you can fix or you need to get someone with more authority.

6. Be truthful. Do not stretch the truth in any way. Your client is hypersensitive when upset, and untruths or exaggerations will exacerbate his frustration and upset.

7. Commit to help and fix the problem, if you can. If you can't, refer to item 11 below.

8. Be sure to ask whether what you have done has satisfied the client.

9. Apologize for the inconvenience caused. Even if the client caused the problem, we are still sorry that it happened and that his experience at the practice was somehow less than expected.

10. Your manager may ask you to call the client later in the week to be sure everything is still okay.

11. If you can't fix it, get someone else who can. Be sure you are selecting the correct individual (nothing is worse to the client than having to tell his story to several different people). The person you bring in at this point should be the "go to" person. If no one is available to address the situation, explain that you want to be sure this goes to the person who has authority to help the client and ask permission to contact him the next time that person is available and have that individual follow up with the client. Then be sure this happens within an appropriate time frame.

Using the Telephone

Many of our first contacts with clients will be on the telephone, and the impression you make when picking up a client's call may mean all the difference to our practice. Remembering the basic principles of good client service discussed in Chapter 3 will help you during your telephone encounters. Not surprisingly, through the tone of your voice, your demeanor transfers to the individual on the other end of the line. Be prompt and pick up the telephone after no more than a few rings—the rule of thumb is that more than three rings is too much—and be friendly and courteous as you accurately record information relayed to you. This chapter outlines basic telephone etiquette, common information you may have to provide over the telephone, and telephone systems in the veterinary profession.

BASIC TELEPHONE ETIQUETTE

Before you pick up the telephone, focus your attention on the exchange you are about to have with your client. Your tone of voice will create the tone of the call. Your client will adopt an attitude similar to the one you offer with your voice. Answer with a smile on your face. Identify yourself to your caller by stating the name of our practice and your first name followed by a question similar to "How may I help you?"

Speak Slowly and Clearly

Remember that the cadence and speed of your voice will affect clients' ability to understand you. Many aspects of veterinary medicine are unfamiliar to your clients, and common veterinary words may be misunderstood by them. Speak slowly and clearly. Learn the value of pauses, waiting for your client's answer or for her to speak first.

Practice speaking with others about the common topics you may be asked to discuss, such as those covered in Chapter 2. Make sure you are comfortable with the subject matter so that you can clearly express yourself.

Listen

Listen attentively to what the client needs. Never assume that you know her question. Be courteous; don't interrupt your client unless absolutely necessary. If it becomes necessary, ask your client's permission by saying, "I'm sorry, Ms. Smith, may I place you on hold for a moment so that I can give you my full attention?"

Be Efficient

Manage your telephone calls efficiently. Your time is valuable to our practice, and your client's time is valuable to her. Be efficient when answering calls. Sometimes you will need to direct your caller in order to maintain efficiency. With tact and friendliness, get the job done. If the client needs an appointment, answer in a friendly manner and ask what she needs. Be friendly throughout the conversation. If you feel the pet's name is cute, for example, say so. However, if the client launches into a complete description of how the pet was named and moves from there into the names of her other pets, you may need to interject a comment that redirects the conversation, saying something similar to "You sure picked a cute name for Sammy, Ms. Smith. Did you want to schedule that appointment for next Tuesday?"

After you have met the client's needs, thank her for the call and be sure to ask whether there is anything else you can help with. Repeat back to the client whichever service you have agreed to provide, saying something like "We'll see you and Fluffy at your appointment with Dr. Jones on Tuesday at three p.m." or "I'll be sure to give Dr. Jones your message." End the call by thanking the client for calling (see SOP 4.1).

USING OUR TELEPHONE SYSTEM

Many telephone systems allow practices to direct incoming calls. If your practice does so, become familiar with where the calls go, who picks them up, and how clients' needs are met. There is a multiple-line system. You have the option to place a caller on hold.

There may be options that allow the caller to choose the area of the hospital she wishes to contact, for example the pharmacy. Your telephone system may take messages when there is no one to answer. Understand this function of the system and who is responsible for retrieving these messages.

The "The Content of Calls" section below will help you figure out how to help clients who call with a variety of common questions and concerns.

Placing Callers on Hold

In general, we do not want to place callers on hold. One of the best ways to make a friendly impression is to personally answer a call. We want to create that impression, so try to answer calls when you are able to help the client immediately. Occasionally, it becomes necessary to put a caller on hold. Always allow clients the opportunity to express their needs before placing them on hold. Saying something similar to "Hello, this is Anytown Animal Hospital. Is it possible for you to hold for a moment or is this an emergency?" Never leave clients on hold for more than a few minutes. Many telephones are set to give a buzz back if a caller has been on hold for more than three minutes. Do not ignore this buzzer. You must at the very least pick up and make sure she is still able to continue holding, or ask for a number so that someone can return her call within a specified time period.

Taking a Message

Our practice has a protocol for message taking. Typically this involves patients recently seen by the practice team, those currently in the hospital, or those with a continuing condition the doctor is treating. You should take complete information from the owner and verify it by reading back what you have written. Ask for proper spelling of the owner's and pet's names. Many names sound similar over the telephone; make sure you have appropriately identified the caller and the pet. Locate the medical record information or chart so the individual responding to the call will have the needed information, and indicate its location with the message (see SOP 4.2).

When and How to Interrupt Doctors

It may be necessary to interrupt a patient appointment to speak with a doctor about a caller. Be sensitive to what is happening in the exam room. If possible, look in a window to be sure you will not startle a pet by knocking on the door. Knock and ask for the doctor. Pass your message and wait to see what the doctor would like you to do. If the doctor is seeing hospitalized patients or is in surgery, attempt to ask her support staff whether you may interrupt.

THE CONTENT OF CALLS

Although the previous sections provide guidelines for all your telephone interactions, callers' needs and the content of the call may create situations that require you to act in a specific manner. The following sections address some of these situations.

Prioritizing Incoming Calls

Sometimes more than one line rings at once or you must deal with more than one situation. Be sure to check with your caller to ascertain her needs. Is this an emergency? Is there another CSR or team member who can answer the telephone? In many practices, there is some backup nearby for the CSR on telephone duty. Once you have determined why the person is calling and ensured that the most pressing calls are dealt with first, you can help the caller. Refer to Chapter 5 for clients who are calling to make an appointment.

Giving Advice

No matter how skilled you become at your client service duties, there are limitations to the types and amount of information you can give out to your clients. It is imperative that you refrain from offering any advice that is medical in nature. The only individuals who can make medical decisions and give medical advice are veterinarians. Remember that callers will assume that the person on the other end of the line at the veterinary practice is knowledgeable about veterinary matters. She will think you are aware of her pet's situation and know what is best for the pet. This could inadvertently lead to inappropriate care for the pet. Follow our practice's protocol for callers seeking advice.

The Telephone Shopper

One of your most frequent calls will be the individual seeking information about our services. This telephone shopper creates an opportunity for you to sharpen your people skills and test your ability to paint a picture of our practice. Telephone shoppers don't know anything about the quality of our service or our pet care. At the moment they call, all they know is your voice and the words you say. When clients ask about a particular service, paint a picture of the whole experience. Know our practice well enough to appropriately represent it. Clients will want to know whether we monitor our surgical patients or if a technician stays by pets the whole time they are under anesthesia. They may want to know what kind of vaccines we use and why the veterinarian wants them to provide a fecal sample at annual comprehensive exam appointments.

Be efficient and friendly and provide appropriate information to the new individual. Always offer an appointment for the caller. "I'd be happy to schedule an appointment for Fluffy to see Dr. Jones. Would three p.m. on Thursday the fifteenth work for you?"

The Emergency Call

In every practice, emergency calls will occasionally come through. As discussed earlier, primary to your ability to perform your duties will be your ability to remain calm in these situations. Chapter 2 discussed what might constitute an emergency, but sometimes veterinary emergencies do not appear to be such. For instance, an owner may not recognize the emergency nature of a male cat that is not urinating. The following information will help you recognize some of the less apparent symptoms of an emergency. If you are unsure, ask for help evaluating the caller's situation. Of course, all questions regarding medical care should be directed to a member of the medical team. However, the CSR can be very helpful in directing these calls if she asks a few specific questions that will better define the nature of the call and possibly detect an unrecognized emergent situation. As you ask these questions, carefully document everything the client says exactly as she says it and provide that information to the medical team. You should also be fluent with directions to our practice from all surrounding areas.

If the Owner Reports the Pet Is "Constipated"

"Constipation" can be reflective of actual constipation and straining to defecate, or it can be a symptom of straining to urinate. Urethral obstructions are often misdiagnosed by owners as constipation. Diarrhea can also be mistaken for constipation when an owner witnesses a pet straining to defecate with no progress.

Topics to bring up might include the following:

- **Species of pet.** Constipation may be symptomatic of different problems for cats than for dogs. For instance, constipation is a common presenting symptom for urethral obstruction in male cats.
- **Frequency of urination.** Dogs unable to urinate can also be mistaken as being constipated. This is more true of female dogs, as the posture for urination and defecation can be similar. Some cats may go to the box and act as if they are urinating (straining) but do not produce any urine.
- **Feces production and character.** Small amounts of liquid stool might indicate that diarrhea is the culprit.

- **Pet behavior.** You want to find out whether the pet is bright, alert, and eating and drinking or whether the pet is lethargic and not eating. Cats may become vocal or lethargic as their urination difficulties increase. They may vomit or stop eating.
- **Blood in the feces.** Bloody diarrhea should always be evaluated, especially if the patient is lethargic or not eating.
- **If the stool is dark tar-colored.** Dark tar-colored stool (melena) is indicative of upper gastrointestinal bleeding, as the blood is digested as it moves through the gastrointestinal tract. Generally, this symptom should be relayed to the veterinarian as soon as possible as it may represent an emergent situation.
- **Eating habits and changes.** An animal that is not eating should be evaluated. Appetite is a very good indication of how a patient is feeling at home.

If the Owner Reports That the Pet Suffered Trauma

Trauma of any type may indicate an emergency situation. As indicated in Chapter 2, some symptoms of distress do not develop until some time after the pet experiences the trauma; therefore, asking pertinent questions may be helpful to your medical team.

Topics to address might include the following:

- **Difficulty breathing.** Patients in cardiovascular shock will also have increased respiratory rate and effort.
- **Nature of any wounds or bleeding.** Wounds on the patient's trunk can penetrate body cavities and cause immediate problems such as hemorrhage or difficulty breathing, and future problems with infection and healing.
- **Ability to move.** An animal that has walked is not likely to have a back or neck fracture.

If the Owner Reports That the Pet Has Been Vomiting or Has Had Diarrhea

You might want to bring up the following topics:

- **General behavior.** Knowing whether an animal is lethargic and anorexic will help the veterinarian decide on a course of action.
- **What the pet has eaten.** Has the pet recently eaten anything she normally wouldn't? This question is designed to get the owner thinking about table scraps, different foods, and foreign material. The client may say, "She got into the garbage and ate a corn cob a couple days ago."
- **Pet's age.** If this is a young puppy, then vaccination status should always be acquired.
- **Whether any blood is present.** Blood in the vomitus often looks like coffee grounds as it is partially digested.

If the Owner Reports That the Pet Has Eaten Something

This kind of call can indicate that the pet has ingested a toxin or foreign body. You might ask about the following:

- **Species of pet.** Dogs are affected differently than cats by most toxins.
- **What the pet ate.** When owners say things like "rat bait" or "fertilizer," it is important to prompt them to tell us the active ingredient. Most rodenticides work as an anticoagulant; however, some cause other problems, which are treated differently. When an owner comes in, it is helpful if she brings the packaging of whatever the pet ate.
- **Weight of pet.** Most toxicologic information is based on a milligram per kilogram dose, so we always need to know how much an animal weighs.
- **Medications the pet is taking.** Always get the name of the medication, how many tablets the owner thinks were in the bottle, and the weight of the pet.

4

The best information about the toxic nature of a product comes from an animal poison control center. Knowing the name of the product that has been ingested is vital to determining the correct toxicity.

If the Owner Has Questions About the Birthing Process

Owners with pregnant pets are often inexperienced with labor and delivery of the animal and will call with questions before, during, and after delivery. The information you will need to ascertain to determine whether it's an emergency includes the following:

- **Breed of dog or cat.** Breeds with large heads (e.g., Chihuahuas, bulldogs) will often have difficult delivering and require a cesarean section.
- **Whether the pet is having active contractions.** Dogs and cats should not go longer than thirty minutes in active contraction before delivering a puppy or kitten. Contractions that are lasting more than thirty minutes can indicate a problem with the puppy or kitten in the birth canal.
- **When the pet last delivered a puppy or kitten.** Dogs can go two to four hours between puppies; cats can go four to eight hours and if disturbed can delay labor for up to twenty-four hours. In general, we recommend that if it is longer than four hours since the last fetus was delivered, the pet should be evaluated. Dystocia is much less common in cats but does happen.
- **General behavior.** Lethargy, pale gums, abdominal pain, and weakness can be signs of cardiovascular shock, which can happen with uterine torsion, generally toward the end of gestation, and sometimes while in labor. This is a life-threatening situation and warrants immediate evaluation.

If the Owner Reports That the Pet Is Coughing

Coughing can be indicative of many different health problems, from something minor to major concerns such as congestive heart failure or foreign body ingestion. Asking the appropriate questions can help the veterinarian diagnose the primary cause of the cough.

You might address the following topics:

- **Age of pet.** Older dogs are prone to heart disease and a collapsing trachea, and coughing can indicate a problem.
- **Character of cough.** Is it a soft nocturnal cough, which can be indicative of congestive heart failure, or a dry hacking cough, possibly indicative of bronchitis or "kennel cough?" Or is it a honking cough, which might indicate a large airway collapse?
- **Breathing difficulties.** All animals reported to have difficulty breathing, with pale gray or blue mucous membranes, should be considered an emergency, and the medical team should be notified immediately. Inability to get comfortable, falling asleep standing up or sitting, stretching of the head or neck, and "head bobbing" in cadence with the breathing are all signs of respiratory distress and warrant immediate evaluation.

If the Owner Reports That the Pet Has a Distended Abdomen and Is Dry Heaving

These symptoms can be indicative of the problem sometimes known as "bloat." This is an emergency situation often not recognized by pet owners and should be handled by a trained veterinarian as soon as it's recognized.

Information you might want to ascertain includes the following:

- **Breed of dog.** Bloat frequently occurs in deep-chested large-breed dogs but is not unheard of in smaller breeds.
- **Whether the abdomen is distended.** A distended abdomen is a common symptom of bloat.
- **Is the pet able to produce vomitus or is it a dry heave?**
- **Length of time this has been going on.** The medical team will need to know this information.
- **General behavior.** Is the pet able to walk? Pet owners also sometimes report that the pet is hanging her head and is extremely lethargic.

If the Owner Reports That the Pet Is Unstable, Wobbly, or Unconscious After Being Out in the Sun

This may be a symptom of heatstroke, and the pet's body temperature may be seriously endangering her life.

Questions to ask include the following:

- **Breed and weight of dog.** Some breeds tend to suffer from heatstroke more readily.
- **Length of exposure to heat.** The medical team will need to know this information.
- **Breathing difficulties.** Pets suffering from heatstroke will pant excessively.

Medication Refills

You will receive calls requesting refills of medications. Our practice has a policy on medication refills. Usually it will require that the pet have seen the veterinarian within a specific time frame, typically within the past year. The most important factor is that you get complete information from the caller:

- Owner's name
- Pet's name
- Name of medication
- When it was prescribed
- How the owner has been medicating the pet (i.e., the number of pills per day at what hourly interval)
- Condition for which the medication was prescribed and how the pet is at that moment
- Whether the medication seems to be helping the pet's condition

Many practices ask that you locate the patient's medical record file or electronic data before asking all these questions. So once the client has identified that she is requesting a refill, you might want to say, "Ms. Smith, may I place you on hold for a moment while I get Sammy's chart so I can be sure I understand your request?" Once you have the patient's file, quickly locate the medication that is being requested. If the patient has been seen within the required time frame, gather the information as listed above and let the client know that you will provide the veterinary staff with the information and someone will return her call or have the refill ready at a specified time (see SOP 4.3).

PLACING THE AFTER-SERVICE CALL

A great marketing tool for veterinary practices is the after-service call. You may be asked to place calls after a patient has been in the hospital for services to see how she is doing at home. These calls are a great opportunity for you to bond with your clients. Your supervisor may provide you with a list of patients recently seen by our practice in need of follow-up calls. Typically, these will be routine callbacks after surgery or a recent pet visit. Familiarize yourself with the patient and the services that were provided before placing the call. If you don't understand a service that was provided, you are not the appropriate person to make the callback. When calling, identify our practice and yourself by name. State that you are calling to check in on Fluffy and see how everything is progressing at home. Ask whether the client is happy with the service that was provided, how the pet responded to the medication, and similar questions. Your conversation with the owner should be documented as part of the medical record, whether written or electronic. The important information to record is similar to the information you gather when taking a telephone message:

- Date and time of call
- Person with whom you spoke
- Content of the conversation
- Any information you provided
- If any follow-up is necessary

WHAT HAPPENS AFTER-HOURS

Our practice hours determine the after-hours telephone protocols. If the practice closes in the afternoon or evening, the telephones may be turned over to an answering service or a message system at that time. If calls come in after-hours, you may be asked to return these calls the following day. These return calls should be placed as soon as possible after the practice opens. Your clients will be waiting to hear back from you, and delaying return of their call will look as if you are uninterested in their situations.

If your practice offers twenty-four-hour care, the telephones may be active all night. If you are responsible for the after-hours telephone service, your practice will train you on the services it offers at night. Most calls taking place after-hours are related to pet emergencies, so becoming familiar with the symptoms of pet health concerns will be helpful (see "The Emergency Call" section).

PERSONAL CALLS

Our telephone lines are designated for the professional use of the practice. Please refrain from placing personal calls during business hours. If necessary, during your break time, the telephone may be used for short calls of a personal nature when the need arises. Personal cell phones may be used during your break times. All cell phones should remain off or on vibrate and should be left with your coat or other personal items as you arrive for work.

The telephone is a vital link with our clients for many reasons. The majority of people who visit our practice form their first impression of us during a telephone call. Information vital to a pet's care will be relayed daily to owners, laboratories, vendors, and others concerned with medical care. It is important that you sharpen your ability to collect and provide information during a telephone conversation; asking appropriate questions, responding with suitable answers, and recording accurate information will greatly enhance our ability to meet the needs of our clients and their pets.

CHAPTER 4 SOPs

4

SOP 4.1: ANSWERING THE TELEPHONE

1. Pick up the telephone within the first three rings.
2. Identify yourself and the practice, saying something like "Anytown Veterinary Hospital. This is Lisa. May I help you?"
3. Speak slowly and clearly. Let your voice reflect your smile and your pleasure to be working with the caller.
4. Focus attention on the caller. If you are multitasking, you may miss something.
5. If you are unable to help the caller immediately because you are working with another client, ask whether this call is an emergency, and if not, ask for permission to place the caller on hold. Do not leave the caller on hold for more than a few minutes. Ask another CSR to pick up the holding call if you will be detained.
6. Proceed to answer questions, schedule appointments, or meet the needs of the caller.

SOP 4.2: TAKING A MESSAGE

1. If you need to take a message for another team member, get all the caller's information including the following:
   a. Full name
   b. The company or pet the caller represents
   c. The reason for the call. If the call is regarding a pet's medical condition, ascertain the need so you can tell whether it is of an emergency nature.
   d. The number at which the team member can reach the caller.
2. If the call is related to a medical situation, pull the pet's chart, or locate the information in the computer and attach the message to the file so the team member receiving the message will have the pet's information at hand.

SOP 4.3: TELEPHONE REQUESTS FOR PRESCRIPTION REFILLS

1. Gather the initial information, owner's name, and pet's name.
2. Locate the file or computer record.
3. Locate the information in the patient's record that reflects the medication for which the client is requesting a refill.
4. Verify with the caller the current method by which the client is using the medication. It may have changed since the prescription was dispensed. For instance, the medication may have been dispensed with the instructions to give it every twelve hours, and since that time the owner has changed the way she is administering it to the pet. Questions such as "How are you currently dosing Fluffy with the prednisone?" will help you ascertain this information.
5. Ask for a brief description of how the medication is working. You may ask, "How is Fluffy progressing on the medication? Does it seem to be helping her get better?"
6. Document the information in the pet's medical record, including the date, name of the person requesting the refill, the full prescription information, the response to your question about the medication efficacy, and a telephone number at which the person can be reached.
7. Sign or initial your entry.
8. Place the request in the appropriate place for it to be reviewed by the doctor. This may mean putting the file in a certain place or making a computer note in a certain area of your software.

Scheduling an Appointment

Our appointment schedule allows us to create an efficient service environment in which our clients' personal lives are respected, patients' needs are appropriately satisfied, and our team is able to perform their required tasks without excessive stress. As you can imagine, harmonizing these three elements is sometimes a monumental task.

We have, to the best of our ability, designed our computer software appointment schedule to reflect this philosophy. It is a pivotal part of our daily plan. We schedule more team members to work the busier hours and fewer during the slower times; our doctors perform longer procedures at times scheduled for them to do so, allowing them to pay appropriate attention to pets' more specific needs, such as surgery or advanced diagnostic testing.

It is important for you to understand this philosophy because as you schedule appointments, you will uphold or jeopardize our ability to maintain this delicate balance.

THE BASICS

Typically, clients approach you to schedule an appointment in one of two ways, by telephone (for new clients or new appointments for returning clients) or in person, after they have been seen by the doctor (for rechecks or follow-up procedures).

Orchestrating a patient appointment is much like conducting a musical performance. All the participating individuals need to be proficient at their parts and the whole must come together to create the musical piece. The system works by attempting to predict how much doctor and practice team time a particular patient visit will need. Experience has given us an idea of the time necessary for typical visits. You will learn that we plan a certain number of minutes for a pet's vaccinations and a longer period of time for a surgical procedure, and that the schedule is organized so we can readily see which team members are involved in which procedures. One of our team members will train you on the specifics of our practice's appointment system, including how long appointment times are and what days and times are used for specific appointment types. This chapter outlines the philosophy behind scheduling appointments in a veterinary practice.

Our practice will also provide you with protocols, training webinars or texts, and on-the-job training for the practice management software we use. Keep a small notebook with you during these training sessions to record specific notes that will help you remember the tasks. Ask questions as often as necessary to create your knowledge base of computer software information.

Several veterinary software systems are available on the market. Almost all of them operate on a Windows base and are easy to learn using the point-and-click method of moving throughout the program. You should have little problem learning the system if you are used to personal computer use (see SOP 5.1).

Programs within our computer system are password protected. This means that as you enter a particular program, you will be asked to create passwords to log in. Thereafter, each time you enter this software program, the computer software will prompt you to enter this particular word or phrase that is known only to you. Use of your passwords as you enter various programs identifies you as the individual entering data and recording transactions; therefore, it is important that you keep these passwords private.

Access to the Internet is available at our practice as necessary for our business operations, but Internet access is not available for personal use, communication with friends, shopping, or surfing. An Internet use policy is stated in our practice handbook that you should be familiar with and follow carefully.

GATHERING INFORMATION

Recording appropriate and complete information for each scheduled appointment makes the system run more smoothly. This is your primary task when scheduling for a client's needs. It involves two basic aspects of communication: what the practice needs to know about the client and patient and what the client needs to know about the practice.

The practice needs to be able to accurately identify the client and patient from among the various individuals who use our services. This means you must record the following:

- Client name, address (both physical and e-mail), and telephone numbers (home and cell)
- Pet name, species, breed, and sex

Being this specific is necessary because every practice has several individuals who share common names. This detailed information will tell us which "Fluffy" owned by Tracy Smith we are seeing at that scheduled time.

If this is a returning client, the computer software should allow you to bring up the patient's identifying information. Verify the information with the client ("Mr. Smith, is your address 151 Stark Street in Plains, Pennsylvania? Can you still be reached at 570-292-0877?"), and then schedule the appointment using a client-patient account number.

The practice also needs to know why the client is requesting the appointment, the reason he wants the pet to be seen by the practice. This means you will need to ask the owner about the pet's current needs and, as you grow more experienced, discuss additional services that may be appropriate for the pet. You must record the purpose of the visit as stated by the client. This may include symptoms or what the client feels is wrong with the pet, information from a reminder card sent by our practice, or general client requests. Remember, record exactly what the client tells you, not what you think may be happening with a pet. Accurately recording symptoms helps the doctor determine the patient's history and provide appropriately for the pet's needs. For instance, write that the pet is "scooting on its bottom after a bowel movement" instead of your interpretation of that behavior, such as possible parasites or anal sac problems.

Finally, the practice needs to know the appointment parameters requested or required by the client. You will need to ask the appropriate questions to ascertain the following information:

- What appointment times work for the client.
- Whether he has a preference for a particular doctor.
- Whether the service requested requires a particular date or time (perhaps the practice performs surgery only on Tuesdays). The client, on the other hand, will need to be provided with the following information:
- The particulars about our practice. If this is the client's first visit, he may need to know where we are located, directions to our practice, and, if necessary, any specific information such as the availability of parking. If you have particular marketing pieces that you mail to new clients or a website that provides more information about our practice, you should advise them of those items when scheduling the appointment.
- The specific information about the appointment itself, such as date and arrival time, taking into consideration the need to fill out paperwork or register a patient before the scheduled appointment.

- Any additional information necessary to complete the appointment: Perhaps the client should bring the pet's previous vaccination records (a new patient), or medications need to be given before a particular diagnostic test, or a pet needs to fast before a surgery, or the owner should bring a pet's stool or urine sample to the appointment.
- Any forms that need to accompany the client or that will need to be filled out in advance of the appointment. If forms are available on your website for filling out, let the client know.

Remember, you will be instructed about these appointment specifics as you are trained. Don't be afraid to ask an experienced team member if you are unsure of how to schedule an appointment. The client and patient will be best served if the practice team is able to meet their needs because their appointment was scheduled appropriately.

The Importance of Accuracy

Veterinary practice management software has been designed to create a record-keeping methodology that can build a comprehensive medical record that is both legally viable and financially sound. In other words, the software in our practice is capable of recording the information we need. The responsibility to create that database lies with the team members who perform data entry tasks.

As a CSR, you will be responsible for data entry that will build the foundation of our software system and is very important to our practice. Accuracy is paramount. Incorrect client information, inaccurate patient information, or inappropriate financial information hampers our ability to succeed at our mission. So whether you are setting up an appointment, updating a record during or after an appointment, or taking financial information, take the task of data input seriously.

APPOINTMENT TYPES

Veterinary hospitals typically create several common appointment types for use in their computer software. Knowing the description of each appointment type helps the CSR find an appropriate time for the patient to be seen and evaluated by the veterinarian.

Preventive Health Visits

Preventive health visits are made for pets that are generally healthy but need to undergo routine health care procedures. As you remember from Chapter 2, such procedures may include vaccinations or diagnostic testing. Some of the recommended procedures will be related to the patient's life stage and lifestyle. For instance, as with people, young puppies and kittens receive vaccinations at particular intervals, whereas older pets should have routine diagnostic blood work and radiographs to monitor their continuing health.

Vaccinations must be performed at appropriate time intervals to offer continuous protection from diseases such as rabies, distemper, Bordetella (kennel cough), adenovirus, parvovirus, and other common contagious diseases, depending on geographic locale and other factors. You need to become familiar with the schedule of vaccinations recommended by our veterinarians.

Preventive health visits can be scheduled in advance and with some flexibility. It will be important to harmonize the needs of the client and the needs of the practice. In most practices, these visits typically last twenty to thirty minutes. A new puppy or kitten examination may take longer to allow for review of client education materials. When a client calls to schedule a wellness and preventive health visit, you should ascertain his scheduling needs and review the practice's appointment schedule to verify appointment availability. Our practice may have particular slots reserved for certain types of appointments in any one time period.

Some clients like to schedule as far as six months to a year in advance of their pet's next preventive health visit. Remember, clients will be relying on you to know the appropriate time interval until their pet's next exam, so carefully learn our practice's protocols.

Sick Patient Visits

Sick patient visits are scheduled when pets become ill and are in need of veterinary care. The nature of the pet's symptoms may dictate how you time the appointment. Unless the symptoms require an emergency visit, sick patient visits should be scheduled as early as possible so that they fit into the practice's appointment schedule and accommodate the client.

When a client calls for an appointment and tells you his pet is ill, you need to ask questions to ascertain the nature of the illness (see "The Emergency Call" section in Chapter 4). These questions become vital when you realize that pet owners often do not recognize the nature of a medical emergency. The best way to gain information is to ask open-ended questions such as "*How* is Fluffy acting? *What* are you seeing him do? *When* did all of this start? And *how* was he acting before that time?" The best way to end your questioning is with one final invitation: "*Is there anything else* that you have noticed about Fluffy?" How, what, and when questions allow the client to tell the story and open the door for him to tell you everything that is happening. Asking a closed question that requires a yes or no answer tells you only one small fact. For instance, if you ask, "Is Fluffy urinating?" and the client answers yes, you don't know whether

Fluffy has been in and out of the litter box frequently, urinating a normal or small amount, or the urine has a red tinge to it. Perhaps Fluffy has also been vomiting and refusing to drink water, but the client neglects to include those additional important pieces of information. In pet health care, because the patient cannot describe its own symptoms, it is important to ascertain as much information from the client as possible. Open-ended questions are the key to gathering important information.

Once you have gathered information regarding the patient's symptoms, you will be able to schedule the appointment appropriately, finding your earliest available time slot that fits the client's schedule and provides care for the pet in a timely manner. Summarize the information in the appointment block or the patient's chart so it can be reviewed by the medical team as they prepare for the patient's visit.

Surgical Appointments

Routine surgical appointments are scheduled in a manner similar to wellness and preventive health visits in that they can be planned ahead of time. Types of routine surgical procedures may include ovariohysterectomy (spay), castration (neuter), and declawing. More advanced surgical procedures may be scheduled at your practice or referred to a specialty practice, such as cruciate repair surgery (cruciate injury is a fairly common canine knee injury). You will become aware of the surgeries performed at our hospital.

Surgical appointments should be scheduled only if the patient has previously seen a veterinarian at our practice within the past year. Check with our practice's policies for the length of lapsed time that is allowed.

Clients must follow particular instructions to prepare their pets for surgery. These presurgical instructions should be given to the client at the time the procedure is scheduled. They may include instructions for food, water, and any routine medications the night before the surgical appointment, dropoff and pickup times, and postsurgery instructions.

Emergencies

Emergencies require the veterinarian's immediate help, and patients should be examined as soon as possible. Emergency symptoms such as bleeding, trouble breathing, and inability to urinate will indicate the necessity for an emergency appointment. Refer to "The Emergency Call" section in Chapter 4 for questions to ask clients to ascertain whether they are experiencing an emergency. Most practices have a plan for emergency situations that includes instructions based on whether the client walks in the door with the pet or calls on the telephone.

Remember, when a client calls with an emergency situation, you need to remain calm on the telephone. Speak slowly and in a steady voice. If the client is unable to focus on the information that you need to help him, speak with an authoritative tone. Without yelling, you want to take control of the conversation and say, "Mr. Smith [pause to get his attention], I need some information from you to be able to help you. Are you able to help me gather that information?" Pausing creates segments of conversation and helps the emotional individual focus on what the speaker is saying. Asking a question may also serve to break the runaway monologue that sometimes happens when people panic.

If your practice does not handle emergencies, preferring to send clients directly to a nearby emergency practice, be sure you know the location, hours, telephone number, and other pertinent information for that hospital so you may relay it to clients who call. In this case, be familiar with the emergency practice your hospital uses so that you may reassure clients. They will want to know whether the doctors in the practice are available at all times, if they will have overnight care just as in a human hospital, if they have equipment appropriate for working with emergencies, and similar information. If possible, take a tour of this practice so you will know firsthand what your clients will find when they get to the hospital.

Most practices do, however, see daytime emergencies when they are in the practice. In that case, when the client calls, you should record the client's and pet's names, whether the pet has been at our practice before (so you may locate the pet's medical history), what symptoms the pet is exhibiting, what event has occurred, and how far away they are from our office. If applicable, pull up or take out the medical records and have them available. This will help the medical team get ready to receive the emergency. Be ready with directions to our facility from all the different main roads.

When a client arrives at our practice with an identifiable emergency, you should notify the medical team immediately. Most practices have a paging call that lets the entire team know an emergency has arrived at the practice. You must remain calm, especially if the client is not. The needs of the patient come first. Call for medical team members to assess the patient. When possible, you may want to move the owner to an exam room if he is upset.

As soon as you are able, get the client's information. If the client and patient have been seen at the practice previously, identify the patient's medical history by finding the patient chart or locating the file in your computer system. The patient's medical history may be a vital part of diagnosing and treating the emergency situation. That information should go to the medical and technical team as soon as possible. If the person is a regular client of another practice in your area and the medical history might be pertinent, get that practice's information so you may call them and have the patient's records faxed or e-mailed to your doctors.

Again, reassure the client that your medical team is doing everything possible to help his pet. Speak in a soothing voice but do not give him false hope. Your job during this time is to serve the client by being a voice of calm reassurance and to gather the information our practice needs to work efficiently during this time.

Recheck Appointments

Many times pets need to be seen at follow-up appointments after an illness or surgery. Our veterinarians will indicate the time interval between the initial and follow-up appointments. If this appointment is postsurgical, the time interval may be standard at ten to fourteen days for suture removal. Pay attention to the instructions provided by the veterinarian seeing the pet for the initial visit, and schedule accordingly. Recheck appointments are typically shorter than the initial appointment, averaging fifteen to twenty minutes in length.

Behavior Appointments

Behavior issues are the most frequent reason pets are relinquished to rescue groups or rehomed. You will encounter clients calling for advice with their pet's behavior issues. Some veterinary practices prefer to refer these cases to behaviorists, whereas other clinics will see pets for evaluation. If your practice handles these cases, you should be prepared to schedule appointments. Behavior issues typically take longer to evaluate because of the history the client will need to relay to the veterinarian. Therefore, plan for a longer, forty-five to sixty-minute appointment. Provide the client with strict instructions for entering the practice if the pet is aggressive. You may want the owner to leave the pet in the car, come in and register, and then bring the pet through a side door or through some entrance that allows them to avoid the congested reception area.

Exotic Animal Appointments

Veterinary care for exotic animal species is quite specialized. Typically there are one or two veterinarians in a multidoctor practice who feel comfortable seeing exotic pets.

You should know which doctors see these pets and how they want them scheduled. Your practice may have a separate waiting area or quiet room for these species because they can become stressed by the normal activity in a crowded reception area.

Boarding and Grooming

If your practice has boarding capabilities or is associated with a groomer, there are specific scheduling requirements you will need to learn. Different pets require different boarding and grooming arrangements. The one common point you must be aware of and consistently follow is that all pets coming into the practice for any of these services must be up-to-date (per your practice's vaccination schedule) on all required vaccinations. This may include rabies, distemper, and Bordetella (kennel cough). Some practices may include canine influenza or additional feline vaccinations. Many practices require that pets be free of ectoparasites (fleas and ticks) and have had a recent fecal examination.

Euthanasia Appointments

Working in the client service area of a veterinary practice offers ample opportunity for you to serve people in their time of need. There is no greater service we can perform than to help clients through what might possibly be the hardest moments of their lives. Euthanasia is a gift we are able to give our pets when their suffering becomes too great. Veterinarians provide this service as an expression of their veterinary oath to "use their knowledge and skills for ... the prevention and relief of animal suffering."

When clients have reached a decision to euthanize their pet and call our practice for an appointment to do so, they deserve your consideration and understanding. Practices recognize their need and usually make special accommodations to meet them. Euthanasia appointments may take place in a special room away from the usual exam rooms. Typically there is a more relaxed atmosphere in this area; there may be a couch, a floor lamp that can be dimmed, a rug on the floor, etc. If possible, practices will place this room where the client is able to exit the practice without returning through the reception area.

Appointments should be scheduled to match the client's need whenever possible. The euthanasia may even be an emergency, if the pet is declining rapidly and suffering. Many times, practices schedule these appointments when other activity around the practice has quieted, perhaps at the beginning or end of an appointment block.

It is best to have owners take care of any bill before the euthanasia. Doing so allows them to leave directly after the euthanasia. Your practice may offer cremation or other body care services. These options should be presented to owners before the euthanasia so that all arrangements are made beforehand. Some clients prefer to take their pet's body home for burial. Additionally, the veterinary practice must ask whether the pet has bitten or scratched anyone within the state's rabies quarantine time frame before euthanizing the pet. This can be a difficult question to ask an owner who is inquiring about euthanasia, but it is a requirement. Explaining that you are required to ask whether the pet has bitten anyone within the past ten days (for some states fifteen days) helps the owner understand your inquiry. If the pet has bitten anyone, specific procedures must be followed to ensure that the pet did not have rabies at the time. Our practice will inform you of how to proceed if you encounter this scenario. There may be a place for the client to indicate their answer to your question on the euthanasia form.

Sympathy cards, sent by the practice team, are especially heartwarming to clients who have recently lost a pet. Most practices send cards to clients shortly after their pet dies. You may be asked to participate in this outreach. Be sincere and empathetic in your responses. Also refer to SOP 3.3 on client care during euthanasia visits.

Appointment scheduling is an art and a science. There are many pieces of information to assimilate, such as how long we allow for castration surgery, what information we need to enter into the appointment slot, which doctor has open appointments available on Thursday afternoon, and more. It can seem overwhelming. However, if you follow the basic framework of gathering the information the practice needs to know and providing the information the client needs to know, you will be on the road to scheduling success. See SOP 5.2 for step-by-step appointment scheduling instructions.

CHAPTER 5 SOPs

SOP 5.1: HOW TO ENTER NEW CLIENT INFORMATION INTO PRACTICE SOFTWARE

1. Click on the new client icon (the head icon). A window will open with places for data entry, and the computer will assign a new client number. We do not use the title entry unless there is a professional title such as Dr., so there is no need to enter Ms., Mr., or Mrs.

2. Tab to the first name area and enter the client's first name.
3. Tab through the additional data entry areas and enter the information provided by the client.
4. Always repeat the information you have entered to the client as a method of checking your accuracy.
5. We require that you ask for both a home and a cell phone contact number.
6. Remember to ask for an e-mail address and have the individual sign, allowing us permission to contact him via his e-mail address.
7. Click "Save" before moving on to enter the patient information.

SOP 5.2: APPOINTMENT SCHEDULING

Remember your goal to create an efficient service environment in which our clients' personal lives are respected, the patient's needs are appropriately satisfied, and our team is able to perform their required tasks without excessive stress. Complete the following steps:

1. Find out what the client needs.
   a. Identify the client and the pet. Ask for their information and verify it in the computer system.
   b. Find out what type of appointment the client is seeking.
      - **Preventive health visit.** Schedule these exams for twenty to thirty minutes—during vaccination appointment times, approximately four appointments for each doctor's morning schedule.
      - **Sick visit.** We leave several "sick-only" slots in our appointment scheduler. These are indicated by highlighting. Use these in order, earliest available first, to leave time for people who call later in the day.
      - **Surgical appointment.** Our doctors follow a specific surgery schedule. It is indicated on the appointment scheduler. Each doctor may have a particular number of surgical procedures he can complete during his schedule. Remember that these clients will need to be given presurgical instructions and may have to meet presurgical criteria before their appointment date.
      - **Recheck.** Always try to schedule this with the doctor who first saw the patient for the presenting problem. For minor problems, these appointments may be scheduled for fifteen minutes. You may check the patient's medical record to see whether the doctor has indicated any special instructions for the recheck appointment.
      - **Behavioral consultation.** Sometimes specific doctors at a practice are available for behavioral consultations. These appointments should be scheduled for at least thirty minutes.

- **Euthanasia appointment.** Attempt to meet the client's needs for timing of appointments for euthanasia. Many practices have specific rooms for these services, so be certain the room is available at the time you wish to schedule. We schedule euthanasia appointments toward the beginning or end of the appointment block so that the client is less apt to be kept waiting.
- **Other.**

  c. Ask whether the client has particular preferences.
  - Does the client see a particular doctor?
  - Does the client need a certain day or time?

2. Match the client's needs with the practie's availability.
   a. Look for available appointment times that match the client's parameters and the practice's availability.
   b. Schedule the appointment.
3. Provide the client with the information necessary to make the appointment a success. Give the client all the information needed to facilitate the appointment, including the following:
   - Directions to our practice.
   - How to locate forms that may need to be filled out before the appointment.
   - All preappointment instructions such as
     » Medication instructions.
     » What to bring to the appointment (e.g., a fecal sample).
4. Reiterate all the instructions to the client at the end of the call. Review the following:
   - Day and time of appointment.
   - Name of veterinarian.
   - All specific instructions.
5. Before ending the call, ask whether the client has any other questions regarding the scheduled appointment.

The Appointment Process

Now that you've successfully scheduled an appointment, you need to know how to help clients during routine appointments. As we discussed in Chapter 3, the first impression you make with your clients will set the tone for their visit to our practice and may be the lasting impression they hold on future visits as well. It is best to make the best first impression possible. When a client walks into our practice, make eye contact as soon as possible. As quickly as you can, engage her in a dialogue, say hello, and if you know the client's name or the pet's name, use it: "Hello, Ms. Smith. How is Fluffy doing today?" If you have not met the client before, be sure to introduce yourself. "Hi, I'm Catherine. Welcome to Anytown Veterinary Hospital." Every individual from our practice who works with a client during her visit should introduce herself. The rest of this chapter covers your responsibilities from the moment the client walks in the door to the completion of the visit.

BEGINNING THE CLIENT VISIT

When a client approaches the reception area, you can begin to gather information about the visit as part of your greeting. Adding to the previous greeting, you might say, "Hi, I'm Catherine. Welcome to Anytown Veterinary Hospital. Are you here for a scheduled appointment?" Asking a question draws the client into a conversation that will begin the check-in process.

Because the client is arriving for an appointment, you can use the appointment software to help cue you for the questions you need to ask. Say you open the schedule and see that Ms. Smith is bringing Fluffy for a new puppy visit. You remember that new puppy visits require certain forms to be filled out by the client and that he should have brought a fecal sample along for testing. After greeting Ms. Smith and acknowledging

Fluffy, you might offer a clipboard with the appropriate forms, saying, "Ms. Smith, might I ask you to fill out this information about Fluffy's lifestyle at home? This information will help Dr. Morgan know just what Fluffy might need during today's visit. Do you have a fecal sample with you? If so, I can take that back to the laboratory now, so they can get started on the testing." Always end with an open-ended question similar to "Do you have any other concerns about Fluffy that I should notify Dr. Morgan about before her exam?" This helps jog the client's memory if something other than a behavioral or health issue has come up since she scheduled the appointment.

The most important part of this exchange is that you have clued Ms. Smith in on what will happen next. Clients, especially new clients, feel apprehension as they come into a practice. Although you are very familiar with your surroundings and what happens during a scheduled appointment, they are not. Always attempt to give your clients information about what will happen next during their visit. Perhaps when Ms. Smith finishes her paperwork, you could say, "I can take that information from you, and you may have a seat in our reception area. The nurse will come out and call your name before taking you into the exam room to meet the doctor." All of this exchange makes Ms. Smith feel that you are taking care of her and Fluffy's needs. You are not leaving her on her own to figure out what to do next. If a client is checking in for a euthanasia appointment, you will need to help her through the process. Be alert to special scheduled appointments, such as euthanasia appointments, behavior appointments, and phoned-in emergencies, and anticipate her arrival as much as possible. Refer to Chapter 5 for tips on helping these clients before and during their appointment.

At this point, you should prepare a chart or start a computer record for the client's visit. Be aware of our practice's policies that begin the invoicing process for the client's visit.

Once you have answered all the necessary questions as to the reason for the client's visit, it is imperative that you notify the rest of the team of her arrival. Practices accomplish this in myriad ways. Your practice software may allow you to indicate her arrival, page another team member, turn on a switch, or put a chart into a certain place. No matter the process, be sure you follow through and that the next team member is notified of her presence in the practice (see SOP 6.1).

CONCLUDING THE CLIENT VISIT

Just as your first impression is important, so is your last impression. Typically a lot has happened for a client during her appointment at our practice. The client will have talked to several people, perhaps will have been separated from her pet for a time, typically will have had to wait for service at least for a few minutes, and will have received medical information and perhaps medications or take-home instructions. She may be rattled by all this activity. Helping the client focus on the checkout process, making sure all questions are answered and that he or she has everything that she needs upon leaving, is an important task.

Take time to review with the client all the services that her pet received and any instructions the client has been given and ask whether you have covered all of her questions. This individual attention will be appreciated. If you are the individual finalizing the invoice, make sure the client understands what was done for her pet today as well as what is owed for the services. If you don't understand the items you see on an invoice, ask about them before you encounter them again. You should be able to briefly explain any service or product that is provided to or for a pet. You will not know the medical details of a procedure or service, but you should have rudimentary knowledge you can share with your client if she asks questions (see SOP 6.2).

Collect payment for the services rendered (see Chapter 8). Follow our practice's procedures for recording that payment and providing the client with a receipt. *Always* offer to schedule any future appointments. Even if no follow-up is needed for the day's visit, ask whether the client wants to schedule the pet's next checkup or needed service, and whether she would like to set up other reminders, such as medication reminders. If you do schedule a next appointment, provide the client with a written appointment reminder. This may print from your computer, or you may fill out a future appointment card.

End the conversation with another open-ended question, such as "Is there anything else you need today, Ms. Smith?" Ending with a question allows the client one final moment to review and be sure nothing has been forgotten.

This is a great time to assess how effective our client service has been. Ask the client about the service for the day. "How was everything, Ms. Smith? Did your appointment go as you expected?" If you are familiar with any glitches in the appointment process, take a moment to apologize and explain: "I know we were late getting you in to see Dr. Lee today, Ms. Smith. I'm sorry. She had an emergency surgery over lunch that left her running a bit behind. I hope everything worked out okay for your schedule." If the client has comments about the service or difficulties that arose, make notes and inform your supervisor so that someone may follow up with her.

Always thank the client for visiting our practice: "It was nice seeing you, Ms. Smith. Thanks for bringing Fluffy to see us. Let us know whether you need anything at all." If this was the client's first visit to our practice, be sure you send home a brochure, refrigerator

❝ CSRs have to be alert and respond quickly and appropriately to many kinds of situations. In our emergency hospital, you deal with many emotions in a short period of time. A pet may be critical; the client's upset and emotional, and you need to be calm and efficient. Or a client is making the hard decision about euthanasia; they are sad and scared and need our support. It is stressful but rewarding. The reason for being a CSR in an emergency hospital is to help clients and their pets. They need us.❞

—TAMMY BUDURKA, NORTHEAST VETERINARY REFERRAL HOSPITAL

magnet, or other marketing information to help the client become familiar with the entire range of services we offer.

The best practices make at least one more contact with the client regarding this visit: the follow-up call (see the "Placing the After-Service Call" section in Chapter 4). Calling a home telephone in the few days after a client's visit to ask how things are going and whether he was satisfied with the clinic visit lets the client know you care. The conversation or message can be very simple: "This is Cathy from Anytown Veterinary Hospital. I'm calling to check on Fluffy and to ask whether you were satisfied with the service we provided during Fluffy's visit on Tuesday." This simple service can be an incredible practice builder.

The order of the checkout process may be altered for special types of appointments per our practice's protocols. During appointments for euthanasia, for instance, checkout may take place in the examination room or before the appointment, allowing the client to exit the practice immediately after the pet is euthanized.

––––––

Veterinary visits can be stressful times for clients and their pets, and typically clients' entrance and exit can be the most difficult. Pets are anxious as they enter and in a hurry to leave as they depart. Expediting these transitions is key to the success of clients' practice experience. Beginning with a pleasant greeting and efficient paperwork processing and ending with accurate financial transactions, your expertise in creating a smooth beginning and conclusion to clients' visits will be rewarded by the relationship you will develop with appreciative clients and other members of the team.

CHAPTER 6 SOPs

SOP 6.1: WELCOMING A CLIENT TO AN APPOINTMENT

Remember the importance of first impressions and make the best of this opportunity. You are the face of our practice, and your clients will form lasting opinions about us from their visit with you today.

1. Be prepared for your client's visit. A key component to a successful client visit is the practice's preparation.
   a. Know the scheduled appointments that are due at our practice. Review the schedule frequently. Appointments may be added throughout the day. Communicate with other practice members. If, during a telephone conversation, a doctor advises a client to come to the practice, CSRs should be informed so they know to expect that individual.
   b. Pull charts and create any paperwork necessary for the visit.
   c. If your practice software uses pictures, familiarize yourself with the client and pet due to come in next.
   d. Keep your work area as organized as possible in order to be efficient when clients arrive.
   e. Keep the reception area clean and well stocked with amenities, ready for clients at any time.
   f. Wear a name tag and professional attire, scrubs, or other apparel per our practice's dress code. Be sure you look neat and are ready to be the face of the practice.
2. Exhibit enthusiasm when you see your client arriving.
   a. Acknowledge her arrival, either verbally or with a gesture.
   b. Greet the client and her pet with a smile.
   c. Call the client and pet by name.
   d. If the client doesn't already know you, introduce yourself and make her feel comfortable.
3. Gather the appropriate information per our practice's protocol for the type of appointment that is scheduled.
   a. This may include presurgical authorizations, new client information sheets, etc.
   b. Review the client information on your computer for accuracy. Does the client still live at the same address? Has the telephone number changed?
   c. If the client has brought any samples (urine or feces), offer to send them to the technician for processing.

    d. If the appointment is for euthanasia, be sensitive to the client's feelings. Find a quiet area for the client to wait, away from other clients. Expedite the appointment, as necessary; waiting for an appointment in these circumstances is extremely emotional and difficult for clients. Offer any special amenities that might make the client more comfortable.

4. Inform the client of what will happen next.
    a. Tell the client where she should wait.
    b. Tell the client how and when the appointment will start.
    c. Let the client know whether there is coffee or tea to drink while she waits.
    d. If you are expecting any delay in the scheduled appointment time, let the client know as soon as possible.

5. Inform the rest of the team that the client has arrived for the appointment.
    a. Page the exam room nursing team.
    b. Use the practice's indicators, a switch, charts in a particular bin, or however the system works.
    c. Watch and be sure the team follows up with the client at the appropriate time. If a client appears to be waiting more than fifteen minutes for a scheduled appointment, check on the delay and inform the client about the reason for the delay.

SOP 6.2: CONCLUDING THE CLIENT'S VISIT

Approach the checkout process as an opportunity to reconnect with your client before she leaves the practice. Your time with the client will be the last impression of this visit. She may carry this last impression until the next visit.

1. As a client approaches your desk to check out from the appointment, reconnect with her visually and verbally. Smile and say her name and the name of her pet. "Hi, Mrs. Smith. Are you and Fluffy finished with your appointment?" If the opportunity arises, comment again about her pet: "It is so good to see Fluffy feeling better."

2. Help the client review all the information she has received.
    a. Review the invoice. Go over the line items to see that everything is recorded correctly and that the client understands the charges. If any questions arise, get them answered by the nursing or doctor team before proceeding to close the invoice.
    b. Review the discharge instructions, medications, or instructions the client has received and answer any final questions.

3. Collect and process the client's payment. Provide a receipt for the transaction.

4. Schedule any follow-up appointments. This may be a recheck or follow-up from today's visit or the next regular checkup for vaccinations or wellness and

preventive health procedures. The practice's reminder system may be helpful in cueing this scheduling.

5. Follow up by asking about the service your client received. Questions such as "How did everything go today?" "How was your visit today?" "Was Dr. Jones able to answer all your questions?" or "How was your service today?" and "Did your appointment take place as you expected?" just after the appointment will typically elicit a true response and give you an opportunity to respond to any unmet expectations.

6. Thank the client for using our practice for her pet's health care. "Thanks for bringing Fluffy in today, Ms. Smith. We appreciate the trust you place in us."

7. The order of the checkout process may be altered for special types of appointments.

   a. During appointments for euthanasia, for instance, checkout may take place in the examination room or before the appointment, allowing the client to exit the practice immediately after the pet is euthanized.

   b. Be empathetic, but balance your empathy and sympathy with professionalism. Temper your emotional side and provide service without drawing the client further into the strong emotions associated with a pet's passing.

6

Marketing Our Practice

Marketing is the sum of all the activities we engage in to build a brand, create aware-ness of our products and services, and fulfill a need.[16] Every day we do things to help grow the practice, and so every day we're engaged in marketing. Veterinary practice is a service business; we don't sell a particular object, we sell a service. Clients pay for medical care for their pets. Typically, they do not understand the intricacies of medicine and judge the value of their visit more on the peripheral aspects of their appointment, how friendly we are, whether the practice is clean and comfortable, and whether it is technologically advanced. Clients are not required to seek veterinary care at our practice. They use their discretionary money to seek treatment for their pets and may choose any veterinary practice. Part of the reason you are here is to help create the value that pet owners seek so they will use our practice's services.

Many different things attract a client to a particular practice, and different clients have different criteria for their choices. Every veterinary practice has a style or theme, whether it is low-cost medical care, high-quality service, variety and scope of service, or décor. Clients tend to be satisfied with the veterinary practice that matches their expectations of service style. Our practice has chosen to reach for the stars by offering the best in veterinary care and client service.

Many people find their veterinary practice because of location or referral by some-one who has previously used our services. Word-of-mouth referral is traditionally one of the strongest marketing tools in our profession.[17] People ask others, "Where do you take your pet?" and follow suit. Some psychologists say that it takes about five posi-tive comments to counterbalance one negative comment.[18] If this is true and someone passes along a comment about a negative client experience, especially in today's world of social media, the consequences may be extremely far-reaching. Therefore, we should look at each exchange we have with a client as a marketing opportunity. It is imperative that we make as many good impressions as possible with our clients.

HOW WE MARKET OUR PRACTICE

We draw people to our practice by using the following marketing tactics:

- Branding (having a well-kept facility, website, and social media marketing)
- Personal sales (providing the best care and communicating clearly and effectively)
- Public relations (community event participation)
- Advertising
- Mail and e-mail promotions

Branding

Branding is a marketing term that addresses the various ways in which a business differentiates itself from other similar businesses. Differentiation helps clients decide which practice aligns with what they want and need. Many things, from brochures and websites to hospital décor, qualify as branding measures. All our team members play a role in helping to brand our practice.

Having a Well-Kept Facility

We take great pride in our facility. As we discussed in Chapter 3, it is an influential marketing tool. Clients take in information through all their senses as they enter our practice. They notice the structure of the facility. Whether the structure looks modern may influence clients' impression of the medicine available at the practice. They also notice whether it is clean, whether there is animal hair blowing everywhere, whether the paint on the walls is fresh or peeling, or whether there are urine stains on the rugs. Does the practice smell of stale urine, is there noisy barking or yowling, is the variety of textures used in the décor pleasing or does it appear worn? Are the work areas organized or cluttered and unkempt? All of these structural and environmental factors affect your clients' impression of the practice. We work hard to be sure we present the best impression possible and ask that all our team members participate in keeping our facility a pleasing environment.

As a CSR, you are responsible for the general organization and cleanliness of your workspace and the area in which clients wait for their appointment. Because pets may shed significantly, you may need to sweep the waiting area frequently. Magazines should be kept neat and old issues discarded. Other general cleanliness procedures need to be followed as necessary. (See SOP 7.1.)

Websites and Social Media

When searching for a veterinary practice, many people turn to the Internet. Therefore, the way in which our practice appears online is just as important as the way it appears physically.

Moreover, social media Internet sites such Facebook, Twitter, and YouTube are becoming more popular as avenues through which clients choose a veterinary hospital. Our practice may have a Facebook site to which you can contribute or use to promote our practice.

Personal Sales

Many of our interactions with our clients can be defined as personal sales. These are one of the most obvious marketing techniques used in service-oriented businesses. We persuade clients to comply with recommendations made by our medical and technical team by using verbal and nonverbal techniques. Sales is about building relationships and providing value. Think about it for a moment: When you are happy about a purchase, it is because you feel connected to the service person you are working with or the product you are buying and you understand its value in your life. Conversely, you will be unhappy paying for anything that creates a negative emotion. Connecting with our clients and helping them understand the value of the medical care we provide are a necessity. Personal sales will be a part of many of the activities you participate in as a member of our practice.

7

Providing Excellent Client Service

We hire friendly people and train them well in order to provide excellent client service. As you remember from Chapter 3, we want to greet each client and treat him in a friendly manner. His needs are met as efficiently as possible. We care about his pet's well-being and strive to provide the best veterinary care. This personal aspect of marketing is our strongest advantage, and we want you to be an active part of creating this warm, inviting environment for our clients. Clients who are pleased with their experience at our practice will not only be more likely to take our recommendations for high-quality care and come back for future visits, but will recommend our practice to their friends and family.

Providing the Best Medical Care

Our medical standards are very high. We insist on practicing the best medicine. We hire great doctors and support team members. You can be proud of the medical team you represent.

Communicating Clearly and Effectively

Remember when we talked about client expectations in Chapter 3? We help clients set additional expectations when they call or visit our practice. Good client service is marked by delivering on promises we've made. When we say the doctor will call him, a service will be a certain price, or an appointment will be at a specific time, we help the client set expectations of our performance. If we do not meet these expectations, we will disappoint the client and damage his perception of our practice. Therefore, we all must do our best to promise only what we can deliver.

Additionally, how we say something is many times more important than what we say. For instance, when discussing your client's invoice, talk about the value he received, not the price. Frame the information you offer to him in a positive manner. Discuss the value of patient monitoring when reviewing the surgical price. It is not what you can't do for your client, it is what you can do. If your client asks for payment arrangements and your practice doesn't offer them, you might say, "We offer several options for paying your bill. We accept cash, check, or these major credit cards." If he asks why the practice doesn't dispense medications for his pet without an exam, say, "We want to provide the best care for your pet and that means allowing the doctor to carefully examine her to provide just the care she needs." Chapter 8 includes more tips for talking with clients about money.

Public Relations

Public relations is the act of engaging with the community and sending them a message about our practice. We take part in a variety of public relations activities.

Community Events

We participate in community activities as a service to our community and as an opportunity to be seen by folks who may need our services. You may be asked to take part in these activities. Remember, when you are out at a community event as a team member, you are an ambassador for our practice. Your friendly and knowledgeable manner may be the very reason a client chooses to come to our practice.

Advertising

We use methods of advertising to promote our practice to those who are unfamiliar with us. We use many advertising pathways, specifically print ads, as well as radio and television.

Mail and E-mail Promotions

This kind of marketing is the use of direct channels of communication to reach current and potential clients. Reminder cards are one of the most important means of communication we use as part of our marketing effort, but flyers and other means of direct mail fall under this category.

Reminder Cards

Once we have established an initial relationship with clients, we invite them back again for appropriate veterinary services. Many times we use our computer software to notify owners of these services.

Our software program has a reminder component. It allows us to generate written reminders, e-mails, or postcards most frequently to notify clients of their pet's health care needs. Our ability to contact them is based on the accuracy of the data recorded in our computer system. You will receive instruction on recording and using the computer software reminder system during your training. At this point, we want you to understand that it is a vital part of our ability to provide necessary care to our patients.[19]

A FINAL WORD ON PERCEPTION

We already know that a client's decision to visit our practice or to accept the treatment our doctors are recommending is not based entirely on fact. In fact, studies have shown that clients desire and are driven to make decisions based on many emotional factors,[20] including the bond they have forged with our practice. The study shows they are evaluating the following factors:

- **Accessibility.** Clients want their visits to our practice to be easy. You can make it easier for them by knowing our practice's processes. Study them. Know the SOPs. To the best of your ability, learn how to answer the common questions asked of your team members and be ready to give an accurate answer.
- **Approachability.** Your clients want to feel at home at our practice. You should make personal contact with them. Be friendly; build warmth into your relationship. Give your clients what they need and want. The simple question "How can I help you?" opens the door to client satisfaction.
- **Reliability.** Clients want you to be consistent over time. They want to know that they will get the same service the next time they are in, that their pet will receive care from whichever team member is assigned, and that you will follow through on what you have said you will do. They want to know that the quality of care for their

pet will be superb this time and the next. This is why we follow protocols and have SOPs. Being uniform in our actions allows us to provide consistent quality.

- **Enjoyability and remarkability.** Clients want you to stand out from all the other practices and to know their name and their needs. They want you to wow them so they will feel like posting positive comments on their social media or online review site. By providing excellent service, you help our practice stand out from the other veterinary hospitals in the area.

———

As a service business, our practice relies on the goodwill we create every day. Because people make decisions based on their emotions as well as on the facts at hand, our clients will objectively evaluate the medical care we provide and emotionally evaluate their experience at our practice. Their feelings about our practice, about you, and about your interactions with them will influence their choice of care for their pet. Each interaction that takes place with a client is a marketing moment. As a representative of our practice, we hope you will realize how integral you are to our marketing efforts. In his book *Companies Don't Succeed, People Do,* author Graham Roberts-Phelps states, "Most surveys across industries show that keeping one existing customer is five to seven times more profitable than attracting one new one."[21] We want your friendly nature, skilled help, and compassion to encourage clients to return to our practice for all their pet's needs and to invite their friends to use our services for their pets.

CHAPTER 7 SOP

SOP 7.1: CUSTODIAL CARE OF THE RECEPTION AREA

- Recognize the area for which you share responsibility. Is it just the reception area, or does it include the exam rooms, a restroom, etc.?
- Know which cleaning products are used in which areas of the practice. Where is a disinfectant needed? What is the mopping solution dilution ratio?
- Watch continually for pet hair buildup; with a large dog, it can happen in moments. Sweep or vacuum per our hospital's protocol.
- Dust all areas at least daily. Pet dander builds up quickly.
- Fecal and urine accidents should be cleaned up immediately. Wear gloves when cleaning the area of an accident. Dispose of fecal matter or the urine-soaked cloth in the proper dispenser. Ask a technical team member whether a fecal sample is required for the pet before disposing of feces.

- Straighten magazines and reading material. Dispose of dilapidated, torn materials.
- Stock brochures and client education materials in appropriate areas.
- Wash and clean walls and windows as necessary. They usually get dirtier from dog nose level on down. Your practice may employ a designated cleaning individual; however, if you are noticing dirty areas, so are your clients. Clean these areas as quickly as possible.
- In addition to the client waiting area, keep your workspace and CSR areas clean and organized. Files should be put away, messages put in the proper place, etc. Clients walk in and view your workspace daily. What impression are you making?

7

Financial Information for the CSR

As a CSR, you will speak about and process financial transactions between clients and our practice. And since, as we already learned, there is a psychology to dealing with money, you need to be an ambassador between these two groups. In order to accurately represent the value of our practice's services when speaking with clients, it is important for you to understand some financial facts about veterinary medicine.

YOUR PART IN A PROFITABLE PRACTICE

Veterinary medicine is a service business. We don't sell *things* as much as we deliver service—medical care to be more specific. So when you look around our practice, you don't see stacks of expensive saleable inventory, such as you would at a clothing store or car dealer. However, invoices for medical care are large, and to the uninitiated individual it seems like the practice must be making money hand over fist. Transactions occur with your clients that may be hundreds or even thousands of dollars. It might surprise you to know that in most veterinary businesses, studies show that the majority of every dollar of revenue is exhausted covering expenses.

The two greatest veterinary expenses are personnel and inventory. The practice owners invest more in the people who work at the practice and in the supplies that are used to provide the services than in any other expense they encounter. Although this may seem like it is none of your concern, in your position as a CSR you are an integral link in revenue collection and expense control.

Revenue Generation

As we discussed in Chapter 7, there are financial aspects to your marketing efforts. Studies show that keeping a longtime client may be five to seven times as profitable as attracting a new one. In other words, if a client leaves the practice because of poor service or care, the practice will have to work to gain additional clients to recover the lost revenue. Even if an unhappy client doesn't leave, a satisfied client is more likely to follow the practice's care recommendations and refer new clients.

How well you perform your duties as a CSR has a direct effect on the practice's profitability. You can make a difference in each client's visit to the practice, whether she returns for additional services, and whether she tells her friends about the practice. You are an integral part of the practice's revenue stream.

The practice management has created a fee schedule that allows the practice to pay its expenses and save enough money to meet its future goals while providing the investors a return on their investment. So, as you can see, if appropriate fees are not charged or clients do not pay their bills, revenue declines and it becomes difficult to meet expenses. It is imperative that accurate invoices—invoices that truly reflect all the services provided to pets—are created and that the practice's payment policies are upheld at all times.

Cost Control

The perceived cost of individual inventory items used in a veterinary practice can be deceiving. Medical equipment and supplies are expensive. The tiny screws used in orthopedic surgeries sometimes cost more than twenty-five dollars each. Injectable medications can run into many dollars per milliliter. The monitoring machine that helps save a pet's life may have an initial cost of thousands of dollars. The ultrasound unit, endoscope, or special diagnostic or surgical equipment may cost tens of thousands. Therefore, not only must we treat our inventory like cash, we must also realize the importance of generating revenue in order to pay for our expenses.

Personnel costs are one of the two greatest practice expenses in veterinary medicine. In addition to wages, the practice pays mandated costs such as workers' compensation insurance and unemployment insurance and benefits such as health coverage, uniforms, and continuing education expenses. Therefore, we ask that you use your time at the practice wisely and efficiently. When you see an opportunity to suggest changes that will increase your productivity, discuss them with your supervisor. If you are experiencing downtime and there is work to be done in another area of the practice, offer to help. The ability to use your time wisely is valuable to the practice and will certainly be noticed by those who supervise you.

TALKING TO CLIENTS ABOUT PAYMENT

As we've learned, success in the veterinary profession is dependent on many of the core principles of sales. When a veterinarian examines a patient and determines that health care services are necessary, whether it is vaccinations or emergency surgery, he is only halfway to success in that professional encounter. Beside every patient is the client, and our interaction with that individual is pivotal to our medical success.

Hopefully, by the time the client returns to you to pay for services, the veterinarian will have engaged her and infused an understanding of value for the services that were provided or recommended (i.e., educated the client about the benefits of the services). When that process is done proficiently, the client will return happy to pay for what has been provided. When the encounter has been less than ideal, for whatever reason, the client may be reluctant to pay. Whatever the situation, a good CSR will always seek to create a relationship and increase the client's awareness of value. Remember, it is usually not the price of a service that affects the client's willingness to pay; it is the feeling of value (negative or positive) created by the interactive experience.

There are several things you can do to help show clients the value of the services and products they are purchasing.

Remember the Basics of Great Client Service

Simple actions like focusing your attention on clients, talking directly to pets, sharing a bit about your own pet, and expressing your concern about specific health care situations will help create a connection between you and your clients when they conclude their visit. All clients need to know that you care about them and their pet.

The principle of creating a relationship begins with empathy, and most veterinary professionals, in whatever capacity, come to work with empathy for their clients. We love animals and inherently connect with clients; we understand how important the pet is in the day-to-day well-being of our clients; we *get* the connection. Expressing empathy to your clients creates a caring relationship. It helps them realize that you understand them at an emotional level. They are more than a number in your day.

Understand the Value of the Service Our Practice Provides

If you are unfamiliar with the services our practice provides or if you are new to the veterinary profession, get to know what pet health care is all about. Ask your supervisor if you can spend a day absorbing the routine of our practice's procedures. You will learn what a vaccination appointment consists of, whether our practice monitors its anesthesia patients, what happens during a euthanasia appointment, and more. The more you understand these aspects of our practice, the more meaningful each invoice line item will become to you. Instead of asking your clients to pay for a computer-generated phrase that reads "Comprehensive Physical Exam," you will understand that what you are really asking them to pay for is the veterinarian's knowledgeable review of their pet's medical history accompanied by an investigative hands-on examination and the recommendations born of several years of educational and experiential wisdom. Wow, when you look at it that way, the examination is dirt cheap! When *you* value the services our practice provides and learn how to express that value to your clients, they will value them as well.

Express That Value to Your Clients

There are several easy ways to express the value of veterinary medical care to your clients at the conclusion of their visit. This section lists just a few.

Smile

You would be surprised at the number of studies that have been done on the relationship-building power of a smile. A genuine smile may create a physiological response in the individual who sees it and predispose that individual to smile in return. A smile creates a feeling of well-being, trust, and goodwill—all emotions that should enhance clients' perception of value and make them more than happy to pay for the services provided. Although that may sound clinical, remember that the chain reaction begins with a *genuine* smile. Let your clients know you believe in the services that have been provided to their pet and you understand the importance of their pet's health.

Focus

Focus your attention on the client in front of you during payment procedures. When you are distracted, the client is distracted and does not fully understand the value of his experience at our practice. Many times, multitasking is a necessity; however, when relaying value, focus is necessary. If you want your client to understand what has been provided to her, focus your own attention on the client during your encounter.

Speak in a Caring and Respectful Tone

Our tone of voice, its pitch, cadence, and volume, belies our underlying emotional state. Try telling someone to remain calm during an emergency when you are not feeling calm yourself. Although the meaning of the words you are saying may be "stay calm," your voice will spur the client to excitement. An even pitch and volume accompanied by a steady cadence create clear communication. As you discuss the invoice, speak slowly enough for your client to understand any unfamiliar words; watch her facial expressions for clues that you might need to further explain particular services or products. Ask for confirmation that she has understood the information you have provided.

Provide Estimates and Review Invoices

Whenever possible, review the approximate cost of services with a client *before* they are provided. Most practices use a treatment plan or estimate for services that can be reviewed with the client before the provision of those services. This format of reviewing approximate client costs has been adopted in many service industries and works well in veterinary medicine. As we have said, veterinary medical care is costly and very few individuals have pet insurance; the use of an estimate allows the client to prepare for the costs associated with their pet's visit to our practice.

Review the individual services that were provided. Once services have been provided, a quick review of the items listed on the client's invoice will remind her of the extent of his pet's visit with the veterinarian. This does not necessitate that each line be reviewed but only that the major services or products provided are highlighted. This will also assure you that the client is in possession of whatever products were to be dispensed and that the invoice was created correctly. A simple summary statement or question such as "Today, Ms. Smith, Fluffy was vaccinated for distemper and rabies, her ears were examined, and Dr. French provided some cleaning solution and medication that will help keep them clean so they don't hurt her anymore. Was there anything else that you needed today?" will help the client review the time the veterinarian spent with her pet and assure the practice that everything that was provided has been correctly invoiced to the client.

Clients, in general, do not understand veterinary medical language, and a line item reading "SGPT, ALT, BUN: $75.00" is not going to mean anything to them. A careful explanation reflecting the importance of each line item to their pet's health will create understanding and value. A much more helpful interpretation of the value of that line item is "The doctor wants to run some blood tests that will tell her how well Fluffy's internal organs are functioning. The results of those tests help the doctor know what disease process is affecting Fluffy's body and provide information about the best treatment to make Fluffy well again. The cost of those diagnostic tests is seventy-five dollars."

Don't Prejudge

It is a mistake to prejudge a client's ability or inability to pay for the services we are providing. Whether our opinions are based on past experience or a preconceived notion about this specific client, prejudging will lead to misunderstandings. Expect every client to want the best for her pet and present all the pet health care alternatives available.

Ask Confidently for Payment

"The total of your invoice is $235.50." This statement, spoken with confidence in the value the client has received and in the client's ability to pay, is perceived well. That same statement, spoken with timidity by a CSR who feels it is an exorbitant amount, will generate a negative response from the client. The same words may be spoken, but the reaction will be quite different.

BASIC PAYMENT HANDLING PROCEDURES

As a CSR, it is your responsibility to be sure the practice receives payment for the services provided to the client. This includes ensuring that the total amount due is relayed to the client accurately, that appropriate forms of payment are collected, that the payment is recorded accurately, and that it is secured for deposit into the practice's account.

Most veterinary practices accept cash, checks, and credit cards as forms of payment for services. Rarely, certain clients may be allowed to charge an invoice and pay their account monthly. Your supervisor will make you aware of these special accounts, if applicable, and the standard payment policies followed by our practice. Being knowledgeable about basic financial principles will help you understand your role in the practice.

Confidentiality

Most clients appreciate (and some situations demand) a confidential environment when discussing financial components of a veterinary visit. If a client is applying for credit through a third-party provider or has to make payment arrangements, she should be granted the courtesy of privacy during the discussion. As a CSR, you should be sensitive to the client's feelings and create a private and confidential atmosphere for this type of transaction.

All client financial and personal information must remain confidential. Laws dictate that practices be aware of and protect all personal information. Your computer terminal—which contains client telephone numbers, addresses, and oftentimes more personal client information—should be out of view of other clients and locked down when you are not sitting in front of it. Credit card slips, checks, and other papers that contain financial information must be locked away from public view. Identity theft is a very real threat, and every business is required to protect its clients to the extent possible.

Cash Payments

Cash is still a popular payment method for small business services, and you will handle cash payments at our practice. Because cash creates no paper trail of its own, as credit card slips and checks do, it is important to create that trail as you accept and process a cash payment.

When you close an invoice and accept cash in return, count it in front of the client to confirm the amount she has handed you. Enter the amount on your software payment screen and calculate or observe the software's calculation of any change due to the client. Count the money again as you put it into the cash drawer. If change is due, withdraw it from the cash drawer and count the amount out as you hand it to the client. Always provide the client with a receipt that shows the amount paid to the practice. Because the client has paid in cash, this is the only record of the transaction.

Payments made with cash must be secured at all times. Your cash drawer should remain locked until it is necessary to access it to accept a payment or make change. It is best to keep the drawer in an area that limits clients from casually observing the amount in the drawer. Excessive amounts of cash should be withdrawn from the drawer and placed in the practice's safe or deposited in the bank. Many practices have security cameras that help secure the practice's cash.

Check Payments

Checks are a security risk for the veterinary practice. When individuals write a check, they are asking the practice to believe that they have money in their bank account that will be transferred to the practice when the check is deposited at the bank. In a perfect world, this is a safe way to pay for services without having to carry cash. However, there is no guarantee that the client *will* have money available to transfer when the check is presented. When this happens, the bank notifies the practice that the check is NSF (nonsufficient funds), and the practice receives no payment and must go through many additional steps to try to collect the funds. Sometimes these NSF checks turn into bad debt and collection accounts for the practice.

When accepting a check, there are several steps that reduce the possibility it will turn into a bad debt. Payments by check require careful scrutiny by the CSR. It is wise to follow these procedures:

1. Make sure you are accepting only personal checks that identify the check writer on the check itself. Checks that are not printed with the name and identifying information of the check writer are called "starter" checks. These are typically issued by the bank when a client first opens an account. If they come back to the practice as NSF, there is very little the practice can do to recoup the funds. Most practices do

not accept starter checks. Look to be sure the check includes the name and address of the person writing the check. If the address on the check differs from that in your computer, ask which is correct and identify it in your notes.

2. Make sure the check is made out to our practice. People sometimes confuse our practice with another establishment they frequent. The "Pay to the Order of" line on the check should be clearly written out to our practice, not to a particular doctor or another business. Most practices do not accept second-party checks. These are checks written to someone else and then assigned to our practice as payment. You should accept only checks that are written out to our practice.

3. On the check, the amount to be paid is written in two ways, in numerical format and in word format. Review and verify the amount in numerical and word format with the amount the client owes the practice. It is a common mistake to write the word format as a different number than the numerical format. If this happens, the bank may choose to honor the check for the wrong amount due the practice, resulting in either an over- or underpayment.

4. Double check to be sure the check is dated and signed by the client. Checks should be dated as the date of payment. Having clients date checks for a different date can set up a practice for bad debt. Most states do not allow postdated checks that are written to be cashed at a future time. Some practices choose to hold checks for clients (ask your supervisor about our practice's policies), but even with this practice, checks should be dated the day they are written.

Your practice may use a third-party check verification service. If so, you may be required to run all checks or checks over a certain amount through the verification terminal or place a call to the service for verification.

Credit Card Payments

The most common form of payment at the veterinary practice is by credit or debit card. These transactions are usually easy to process and fairly secure. Practices accept different types of credit cards. Many use primarily MasterCard and Visa services, whereas others also include Discover or American Express. Increasingly, third-party providers are included as payment options for your clients. There is most likely a terminal through which you will process credit card transactions. Transaction methods will be specific to each practice. Be careful to learn and process credit cards according to our practice's payment policies. Accurate data entry is vital during credit card processing. Entering wrong amounts, processing under the wrong card type, or creating a sale when you meant a refund can cause major delays and hassles for your team members and clients.

Each of these card transactions costs the practice money. Credit card–processing companies typically charge the practice a percentage of the sale that is run through the card and may also assess additional fees for each transaction. This means that accuracy on your part—entering the correct amount of the sale, swiping the card versus entering the numbers by hand when possible, checking the expiration date—will be helpful money-saving steps.

Credit card theft—an increasing problem in our society—has prompted regulations governing the security involved in processing credit cards. Businesses are required to keep credit card information as safe as possible. Much of a client's information and credit card numbers must be kept confidential. In order to watch for credit card theft, you should always verify that the name on the credit card is the name of your client. If the client says that she is authorized to use another individual's card, you should call and verify that with this card owner.

If your practice accepts credit cards over the telephone, verify the card owner's mailing address and security code on the back of the card. Enter this information into your client's record in some manner for future reference, if necessary. It is not wise to include a client's credit card number in her pet's file. Most practices refrain from storing credit card numbers for their clients.

Pet Insurance

The number of clients with pet insurance is increasing. Typically, practices require payment from the client at the time the pet is seen and then provide the client with the necessary information to submit the claim. The client receives the reimbursement from the insurance company. Check with your supervisor to better understand our practice's policy on pet health insurance so that you can accurately instruct your clients.

ACCOUNTS RECEIVABLE

Let's take just a moment to address the situation of nonpayment by the client. Because of the tight margins in today's veterinary practice—remember, most of each dollar earned goes toward paying expenses—practices have generally adopted policies that require payment in full when services are performed. There may be the rare instance when the practice extends credit to a longtime client who has difficulty paying an invoice in full or in a Good Samaritan situation. These situations should be handled by your supervisor.

Hopefully, your clients are prepared in advance for the cost of the services they have received. Most practices use treatment plan estimates that indicate the recommended services and the associated costs to the client before providing the service for the pet. Using estimates and asking for deposits on surgical or other expensive procedures prevents the client from being surprised by a large invoice.

So what do you do when a client says she doesn't have money to pay the invoice in full? As a new team member, this can be tricky. You should always involve your supervisor in these situations until you are told you can present the options yourself. And there are options other than letting the client leave without paying.

Remember what we learned about the importance of expressing the value of our services and being compassionate and caring but also firm when presenting invoices? Payment options at your disposal include letting the client call a friend or relative who can provide a credit card number over the telephone, helping your client apply for third-party financing, offering to hold the pet in your boarding area free of charge while she goes to her financial institution, and offering to hold a check (if practice policies permit). At the very least, do not give the client take-home medications and other outpatient and nonessential services if payment will not be received. The practice incurs costs for all products and services for which we should be paid. If practice policy allows, provide a prescription for medications instead, which allows the client to purchase the medication at a human pharmacy at lower cost.

Financial transactions can be stressful to clients at a veterinary practice and to members of the team, but we would not exist without receiving payment for our services. Understanding the value of the services we offer and the best methods of presenting payment options to our clients (see SOP 8.1) will help you become more comfortable in your daily responsibilities. Remember to keep all client transactions confidential and follow our standard payment procedures at all times (see SOP 8.2).

CHAPTER 8 SOPs

SOP 8.1: PRESENTING FINANCIAL INFORMATION

- Remember that your demeanor matters.
  - » Smile—it's catching.
  - » Focus your attention on the client. No matter what is happening around you, you must focus on the client in front of you to effectively present financial information.

» Be confident. You are responsible for understanding the services you are talking about and their value in the client's and pet's lives. Observe our practice's medical procedures and have an experienced team member explain them to you. Practice what you will say. Role-play with your supervisor or other team members and learn to explain to clients the services that have been provided for their pet. Know and be able to express the value of our practice's services. Speak slowly and clearly. Medical jargon is difficult for the average client to understand.

- Provide financial services in a confidential setting.
  » Speak with the client in a separate room, perhaps the exam room, about any confidential matters.
  » Keep all financial records from view by the general public.
  » Do not keep extraneous client personal financial information at the practice.
- Provide estimates for service and future treatment plans.
  » Review these with the client before providing services.
  » Speak with confidence about the medical necessity of all the proposed procedures.
  » Ask for confirmation that the client has understood.
  » Secure a signature on the written treatment plan, including an estimate.
- Review invoices.
  » Review each line item or review a summary of the services provided (our practice has a preferred protocol for this procedure).
  » Speak with confidence about the medical necessity of all the provided procedures.
  » Ask for confirmation that the client has understood.
  » Ask whether all the client's and patient's needs have been met.
  » After you are sure the client is satisfied, explain the total amount due for services.

SOP 8.2: ACCEPTING PAYMENT

- Cash payments
  » Count the cash in front of your client after she hands it to you. Count it again as you put it into your cash drawer. Count change as you take it from your drawer and as you hand it back to your client.
  » Keep your cash drawer secure and out of sight of the general public.
  » Always provide your client with a receipt.
  » If money above our practice's cash drawer limits accumulates in your cash drawer, report it to a supervisor so cash can be removed to the practice's safe.
- Check payments
  » Be diligent; if your practice will get stung with a payment loss, checks are the most frequent offender.

» Do not accept checks unless they contain the client's entire identification information, including name and address.

» Verify the check information. Are the amounts in the numerical and word lines the same? Is the practice's name correct in the "Pay to the Order of" line? Has the check writer signed correctly? Is the date correct? Does the amount on the check match the amount due the practice?

» Stamp the back of the check with the practice's deposit stamp.

» Secure the check in the cash drawer.

- Credit card payments

» Verify that the name on the credit card matches the client's identification.

» Run the card through your card reader.

» Verify the amount due the practice with the amount you are entering into the card reader.

» Present the machine receipt to the client for signature and secure it in the cash drawer. It is often helpful to write the client's account number at the top of the receipt.

» Provide the client with her copy of the credit card receipt and a receipt generated from your computer.

- Accounts receivable

» If your practice provides a billing option to particular clients, become familiar with all the necessary steps in the accounts receivable protocol.

Medical Records

A medical record is a compilation of all the practice's information about a patient. It includes the client's information, the pet's identification, the veterinarian's notes regarding medical care for every visit to the practice, any medications provided, which diagnostic tests were performed and the results of those tests, communications with the client by telephone or other means, and a list of the pet's diseases, surgeries, or other procedures and the signed consent forms for those procedures. The information that is placed in the pet's medical record creates an outline and a timeline of the pet's medical needs. Many clients bond to specific veterinary professionals, and so the medical record may contain facts relating to the pet's life from youth to old age. Keeping a comprehensive medical record for every pet seen at the practice is an important client service responsibility. The practice's medical records, while documenting patient information, also drive several vital aspects of the practice's life, including the quality of patient care, the practice's overall financial health, marketing capacity, regulatory and legal compliance, facility management, and team member satisfaction.

Although it is not necessary for you to understand all these aspects of medical record keeping, knowing the value of a medical record will help you complete your medical record-related tasks with the accuracy desired by your supervisor and the practice management team and will help you succeed at the practice.

THE IMPORTANCE OF MEDICAL RECORDS

A pet's medical record is seen as a legal document. As such, it may be subpoenaed for use in a legal proceeding. Actions such as standard of care inquiries by the State Veterinary Medical Board or a private court, specific procedures or service inquiries by local tax authorities, purchase and legal use of controlled substance inquiries by the Drug Enforcement Agency, drug use inquiries by the U.S. Food and Drug Administration, as well as other actions of government agencies may initiate scrutiny of a pet's medical record. Diligent preparation of the medical record may make the difference between a positive and a negative outcome of these inquiries for the practice and its veterinarians.

A separate medical record must be kept for each pet and must always be readily accessible. This means that a member of the practice team should be able to locate a record in no more than twenty-four hours' time. If you are the person entering data into a computerized medical record or filing a paper copy medical record, how you enter the data or where you file that chart is a vitally important aspect of your daily duties.

Any entry into a medical record must identify the individual who recorded the entry. Whenever you record a client's conversation or add data to a record, your name, initials, or another identifying code must be included with the entry.

The information contained in a medical record is confidential. You should not release medical record information to anyone without checking with your supervisor. He will know the appropriate response to an inquiry for medical record information. Be familiar with our practice's specific protocols for this process, including the use of medical record release forms and consents that require that the patient's owner sign for the information to be released to a third party.

As stated above, all aspects of the patient's care must be recorded. For instance, examination reports, diagnostic testing results, signed owner consent forms authorizing treatment for procedures, a list of services provided and their costs, and communications with the owner should be included. Our practice has defined the process of recording this information for pets seen. Your responsibility is to learn that process and diligently carry it out each day, maintaining the appropriate information in an easily retrievable manner.

HOW PRACTICES USE MEDICAL RECORDS

Obviously the most important aspect of the medical record is that it contains the pet's medical history. It creates the "story" of the pet's medical treatment, including vaccinations, illnesses, surgeries, and other events. Veterinary practices record and review all these entries in accordance with their standard of care, to ensure that each patient gets the best medical service. If the pet is of age for particular vaccinations, it is important to know whether previous vaccinations have been given in a timely manner. In order to provide consistent, appropriate care, the veterinarian must frequently refer to the pet's medical history. If the pet presents with symptoms of a disease that affects the liver, for instance, and the current blood profile shows elevated liver results, it will be important to know whether previous results were within the normal range. If a pet is exposed to a disease that can be prevented by vaccination, it will be important to know whether that pet has been vaccinated. Many such examples exist for every patient seen by the practice.

In addition to documenting the pet's medical history, the medical record may be useful to the practice for generating revenue, evaluating productivity, and tracking inventory. For instance, you may be trained to review a pet's medical record before his visit to the practice to ascertain whether the patient has been optimally vaccinated and has undergone required recent diagnostic testing or medical procedures. This aspect of medical record review is sometimes called compliance review. It can be instrumental in giving the pet the appropriate medical care associated with his stage of life, as well as in productively using the resources of the practice.

You may also be included in our practice's medical record auditing procedures. These involve comparing the pet's medical history with the practice's invoicing software program to identify areas where charges are being missed or misapplied. Whatever the practice's medical record protocols, you are instrumental in maintaining this vital practice resource.

ACCURACY IN MEDICAL RECORDS

We've already discussed the importance of accuracy. Once you understand the multifaceted use of the patient record and the legal nature of its documentation, the necessity of accuracy in medical records becomes abundantly clear. This includes accuracy of data entry and the need to update information on a regular basis. A client's personal information may change rapidly. People are mobile; they change addresses, telephone numbers, jobs, and partners during the course of their association with our practice. Much of the responsibility for updating information in a patient's medical record is assumed by the CSRs.

When a client calls or appears for an appointment, you should verify the information that is currently recorded in the patient's medical record. Ask whether the client's address has changed, whether we are able to reach him at the same telephone numbers, and whether we may also speak with the other individuals listed on the medical record about the pet's care. All these questions should be reviewed each time you interact with a client. When you enter information, it is essential that you write legibly or type accurately. Take a moment to review your entry to be sure you have all the information correct.

A patient's vaccination history is vital health information, and sometimes clients are mistaken about where and when vaccinations were administered. When working with a new client who provides you with a verbal medical history for his pet, it is best to ask whether you can verify the vaccinations by calling the previous veterinary office and asking for vaccination records. Always ask for any updated vaccination history when a pet has not been at our practice for a period of time. Clients may be seen at more than one veterinary office and receive vaccinations elsewhere.

Medical Record Audits

Because creating a complete and accurate medical record is so important, our practice engages in medical record auditing procedures. After you have become familiar with our medical record systems and are accurately recording information, you may be asked to help in this process, which consists of comparing the pet's medical record and the client's invoice with our approved standard of care. This process helps us determine whether the pet is getting all the recommended procedures appropriate for his present age and state of health as well as helping determine the correct entry of invoice charges (see SOP 9.2).

A pet's medical record is a legal document, and everything entered in it can become part of court proceeding. The medical information it contains is pertinent to the pet's care. As a CSR at our practice you are one of the keepers of this vital information. We have strict guidelines for processing the data we collect in our medical records and expect that you will follow them accordingly (see SOP 9.1).

CHAPTER 9 SOPs

SOP 9.1: MEDICAL RECORD DATA ENTRY

If the patient has never been seen at the practice, follow the steps listed below:

1. Ask the owner for the medical history. If it is available, you may verify the accuracy of the information it contains and use it for data entry into your system. If the client has no medical history for the pet, ask whether you can contact the previous veterinary office for copies of the pet's medical history. If the patient is a puppy or kitten, there may only be the record from the breeder, or no record at all.

2. Gather and enter appropriate client information and pet information in the practice's medical record, whether it is a computer or a paper form entry. In addition to name, address, and telephone number, you may need to ask the following questions:

    a. "Is there another person you would like to list on the account whom we may contact in regard to Fluffy's care?"

    b. "How do you spell Fluffy's name?" (You will be surprised at the way people spell their pet's name, and it is important that we spell it correctly.)

    c. "Are there any additional telephone numbers at which we might reach you?"

3. When the client comes to the practice for an appointment, ask him the reason for the visit and record it in the patient's medical record. This should be a simple statement like "First puppy visit" or "Shaking his head." Once the client states his primary reason for the appointment, you may want to ask whether there are any other concerns regarding the pet's care for the doctor to address, and note these as well.

4. Be sure you are identified as the individual who entered the information into the medical record. If you are creating a paper record, write your initials or identifying numbers at the end of the entry. If you are entering information into the electronic medical record, be certain the login identifies you appropriately.

If the patient has previously been seen at the practice, take the following steps:

1. Verify the previously recorded client information. Ask questions about the contact information and individuals listed on the account.

2. Verify the patient's information, asking a question like "Has anything changed in Fluffy's medical history since she was in last September?"

3. Review the information listed on the pet's vaccination record, problem list, and medications list. If items look as if they don't match your vaccination schedule or might require updating, alert a technical team member so that she may ask the client about it at the beginning of the appointment, or, if you have been trained to do so, ask for more information from the client.

4. Ask the reason for the visit and if there are any other concerns.

5. If you are adding any information to the record, make sure you are identified appropriately.

SOP 9.2: AUDITING MEDICAL RECORDS

After a client appointment, review the medical record alongside the invoice and in light of the practice's standard of care protocols:

1. Print the client's invoice.

2. Compare the information entered into the medical record with the procedures that apply to the client's invoice. See whether charges were entered on the invoice for all the procedures performed, administered, or received and any products that were sent home with the client after the appointment.

3. Determine whether the services were offered in accordance with the standard-of-care protocols for our hospital. The standard-of-care protocols may include our vaccination schedule, deworming protocols, and laboratory or other diagnostic testing schedules.

4. Note any discrepancies and call them to the attention of your supervisor.

Safety for the CSR

The Occupational Safety and Health Administration (OSHA) has created regulations to help protect American workers. The veterinary profession falls under these regulations, and our practice has protocols designed to protect you and other team members. In addition, the American Animal Hospital Association (AAHA) has created protocols for veterinary team member safety. You should become familiar with the entire safety program developed by our practice. The items mentioned here are just a few of particular interest to client service team members.

In addition to safety issues common at any workplace, there are specific safety issues inherent in the veterinary profession of which you should be aware. These include animal bites, zoonotic (animal to human) disease transmission, ergonomic injuries, evacuation protocols involving pets, and veterinary product safety information.

One of the most prevalent reasons why new team members seek employment in the veterinary profession is a love of animals. On a daily basis, cute pets will arrive in our practice. Knowing some basic animal-handling safety protocols will help you avoid pet altercations that result in injury.

AVOIDING ANIMAL BITES

Most animals that enter the veterinary practice are under some form of stress, either from illness, injury, or just the unusual medical environment. As such, pets that are typically friendly and outgoing may be wary and edgy. As a rule of thumb, it is best to avoid reaching out to or trying to pet an animal as it presents in the practice. Pets may feel the need to protect their owner or themselves and snap, snarl, or swat at you. As you proceed through your training and tenure at the practice, you may come to know some of the common overt signals of pet distress, for example ears laid back, hair raised, and stiff body posture; however, the unpredictable pet is always a possibility and it is your responsibility to protect yourself and others. Do not attempt to physically interact with a pet as it enters the practice and approaches the front desk.

When you are visiting in the treatment and ward areas of the practice, do not reach into cages or attempt to touch pets that are being examined or undergoing procedures. A pet may react to pain by snapping or biting. Some don't like being held tightly for procedures and may react out of stress. Some don't like being in a cage and may be aggressive to anyone who approaches the kennel area. Technical team members working with pets will have a much better grasp of a patient's status, so you should always check with them before interacting with a pet.

ZOONOTIC DISEASES

Zoonotic diseases are diseases that can transfer between different species. Several animal diseases may transfer to humans. From common treatable diseases like round-worms to the fatal, less common rabies, these diseases pose a threat to the veterinary team. Information about the transmission pathways associated with these pathogens will help you protect yourself from infection.

Rabies is transmitted through the saliva of an infected animal, usually by a bite. You may never encounter a rabid animal at our veterinary practice, but any unvaccinated pet is suspect, especially if she is presenting for neurologic symptoms. Avoid placing yourself at risk by handling stray or unvaccinated animals. Avoid bites by carefully following our practice's animal-handling protocols (see above).

There are some parasites that humans can pick up through other forms of contact with animals. Roundworms, for instance, are transmitted by ingestion of roundworm eggs. Although we don't think we are exposing ourselves to these microscopic eggs, our activities at the veterinary practice may put us at risk. The primary protective method to prevent such transmission is use of examination gloves whenever handling feces and frequent hand washing after pet handling and before eating and drinking. Food should never be consumed in patient treatment areas of the practice. This activity is regulated by OSHA and AAHA and simply makes sense for protecting yourself from pathogens. Our practice has developed specific infectious disease control policies of which you should be aware and through which you may protect yourself.

ERGONOMIC SAFETY

Every workplace has its own particular ergonomic challenges. Those typical to the veterinary environment include repetitive-motion injuries associated with computer data entry and lifting injuries from pet handling situations. You should seek the advice of your supervisor for the methods our practice has instituted to prevent such injuries. Lifting heavy objects with help or proper devices, varying your work posture, getting up from the computer and filing for a while, and moving the keyboard to a more comfortable position for long periods of typing are precautions with which you should be familiar.

FIRES AND OTHER DISASTERS

During your orientation and initial training, you will become familiar with our practice's evacuation protocol. If you don't know where the designated assembly area for emergency evacuation is, you should find out now. In the event of a fire, natural disaster, or other hazard that necessitates evacuation of the practice, you should be aware that you are required to exit the practice in a manner that protects human life. This means that you will help clients exit safely and do so yourself. You should never return to the evacuated building to try to rescue hospitalized pets. Instead, sound the alarm, evacuate the practice according to procedure, and notify professionals. Our practice has developed protocols to address patient safety in these situations, and professional rescue workers will be more able to safely evacuate animals than any of us will. Some natural disasters come with a warning, but you should still be aware of our practice's procedures in the event of a blizzard or similar disaster.

HAZARDOUS CHEMICALS AND PRODUCT SAFETY INFORMATION

Some products used in the veterinary practice may be hazardous. Every team member should be aware of the location of product safety information and how to react to accidental product exposure. If you haven't already, locate our practice's product safety information catalog and become familiar with the procedure of identifying a product and understanding its hazards.

SAFETY IN THE RECEPTION AREA

Several safety issues may develop in the client service reception area, including a slippery wet floor, pet altercations, distraught client actions, or veterinary medical emergencies. As the CSR, you are responsible for overseeing this gathering area for your clients and their pets, and you must remain alert to situations that require your intervention. Be aware of the possibility of an aggressive altercation between pets in the client waiting area to help keep your clients, their children, and their pets safe. All clients should keep their pets on a short leash or in a carrier when they are at the practice. Although this may seem apparent to you and me, it is not to some owners who consider their pets docile friends. If you see a client allowing her pet to roam freely or on an extended leash,

10

politely ask her to collect her pet and keep her close by. To avoid offending owners, let them know that although their pet may be friendly, another pet may not be and that you are protecting their pet from fright and injury. If you see children wandering and approaching pets other than their own, speak to the parents and advise them of the risk and need to keep their children safe. When it seems impossible to maintain a safe client service area because of specific conditions, for instance an aggressive pet or unruly children, it is best to direct the offending client to an exam room and ensure the safety of all.

Unfortunately, we also must be aware of the possibility of violence in our practice. In our society, it is not uncommon to hear of attacks by disgruntled clients, estranged spouses, and criminals. Because we keep cash and controlled substances on hand, there is a risk of burglary or other violence. If you feel threatened and no one around is around to help you, exit the area and seek help. If necessary, call the police. A panic button at the CSR desk will summon the police.

Patient safety is a primary concern for our practice. In addition to watching for pet aggression in the waiting area, we want our CSRs to watch for emergent health conditions. Be aware of the general countenance of patients waiting for appointments. If clients are distressed by their pet's current condition, or you become aware of declining pet health, immediately call for a member of our medical team to assess the pet. We pride ourselves on creating a safe practice for our clients and their pets (see SOP 10.1).

Safety in the veterinary hospital must be the concern of all team members. All work environments hold challenges, and ours is no exception. Dog bites, zoonotic diseases, and hazardous chemicals are common threats. It is your responsibility to work in a manner that protects you, your clients, and your teammates. Please become familiar with our practice's safety protocols and diligently follow them. If you become aware of a hazard, immediately inform your supervisor so that we may correct it.

CHAPTER 10 SOP

SOP 10.1: CONTROLLING THE RECEPTION AREA

No one else in the practice can visualize the client reception area as well as the CSR. Therefore, it is your responsibility to police the facility, clients, and patients in the vicinity at all times. Client safety and comfort should be your primary concern.

- **All pets should be leashed or crated as they come into the practice.** If a client arrives without proper pet restraint, be prepared to provide it with a smile and simple statements like the following: "Ms. Smith, I'd appreciate it if you could put this leash on Sally. She is very friendly, and we wouldn't want her to accidentally approach another less friendly pet and be injured." "Ms. Smith, I have a carrier you can use for Fluffy [single-use cardboard] while you are waiting for the doctor. It will keep her safe. I worry that she might run out when the door is opened."

- **Stressed pets will often act out and behave aggressively.** Veterinary hospitals are typically stressful places to pets. They may act fearful (attempting to hide behind their owners) or aggressive (laying their ears back, vocalizing, or raising their hackles). If your waiting area is crowded, this type of behavior is more likely to manifest itself. If your reception area is becoming crowded, seek help from another team member. Perhaps someone can wait more safely in an exam room.

- **Excited children may overstimulate and agitate pets.** Children in a crowded waiting area are a challenge you must face. If a client's children are approaching strange pets, making loud noises, or moving erratically and their parent is not taking appropriate steps to protect them, you will need to act. Check to see whether the family can be moved to an exam room; offer books or other kid-friendly items our practice has available. If all else fails, approach the children directly, saying something like, "Hi, I'm Sally and I work with the veterinarians here at the hospital. I need to ask you to sit by your mom and keep your pet comfortable. We have lots of pets from other families here today, and they aren't used to all this activity. It is frightening them. We should be able to get you in to see the doctor very soon." *Most* clients who are not already controlling their kids need and welcome your help if it is presented in this manner. You may also directly approach clients and ask them to step in for similar reasons.

- **Watch for spills, soiling, and tripping hazards.** With anxious pets eliminating on the floor, people spilling drinks, and leashes draped across the floor, the client reception area can be a minefield of obstacles. Keep an eye open for these hazards and correct them immediately. Remove urine or feces to a garbage can where the odor will be contained.

- **Keep the area neat and clean.** Whether it is your responsibility to clean it or simply to notify others that it needs to be cleaned, the reception area is your domain. Act quickly to clean up or straighten up. Remember that clients don't see all the treatment areas of our practice and will form opinions about our medical care based on the cleanliness of the entrance and reception area.

10

- **Monitor your clients' wait times.** You are the guardian of clients' impression of our practice. In this day and age, nothing aggravates a client more than waiting to be seen. Decreasing waiting time is imperative to providing good service. If a client has waited longer than fifteen minutes, contact a team member working with the pet and let her know. Follow up to be sure the client is informed of the reason for the delay.

- **Observe pets in the reception area; if you see any symptoms of declining pet health, immediately call for a technician to assess the pet.** Sometimes clients wait until the last minute to bring a pet to the veterinarian. They schedule a sick visit for a pet that may need emergency care. Therefore, their pet may experience a health crisis while waiting to be seen. Watch for seizure activity, loss of bowel control, salivation, panting, pacing, or other symptoms of distress. Monitor clients' level of concern. Clients may feel uncomfortable approaching you to tell you they need help; however, if they are becoming more concerned about their pet, you should be also. If you or the owner is concerned, ask a team member to assess whether the patient needs immediate assistance.

CHAPTER ELEVEN

The More Advanced CSR

The SOPs in this text have been directed largely at the new and learning CSR, although we have also introduced more advanced concepts. The following charts are designed to help you see the natural progression of growth in our practice. Each level described is recognized as carrying more responsibility in the CSR department. Your supervisor will provide guidance and training as you move from one level to the next. Although general time references are included for each level, we understand that you may progress more quickly through these training levels.

FIGURE 11.1   Level 1 Characteristics

The new CSR should be able to fulfill the following primary work responsibilities. They encompass client service basics, fundamental veterinary knowledge, and familiarity with our practice.

General

- Is friendly and warm to all clients and team members
- Maintains a positive attitude throughout the workday
- Displays good work habits (i.e., punctual, present, appropriate appearance)
- Understands and adheres to practice employment and client service–related policies

Communication

- Knows species, common breeds, and general veterinary terminology and uses them appropriately in conversations with clients
- Clearly communicates travel directions to the practice
- Understands and can review all forms used in the practice
- Understands and can explain major CSR-related policies in the practice
- Answers telephone and provides telephone-related services appropriately, such as taking messages and noting medication refill information

Computer

- Accurately creates software data entries related to CSR functions
- Schedules regular appointments accurately and provides clients with appropriate appointment-related information.
- Understands software invoicing operations and provides accurate financial transactions, reviewing with clients as necessary
- Understands personal end-of-day procedures for reconciling transactions

Medical Records

- Understands the legal nature of the patient's medical record
- Understands and provides client confidentiality
- Knows the format for the practice's medical records
- Knows all forms associated with the patient's medical record
- Understands the practice's medical record flow
- Easily finds and appropriately files or stores patient medical record information

Operations

- Knows and follows basic safety regulations relating to the practice and the CSR position
- Keeps the reception area clean and tidy, cleaning up "accidents" quickly and organizing the CSR workspace as required; notices when supplies are running low and alerts appropriate individual
- Operates computer and other office equipment correctly

Financial

- Understands basic practice economics, including cost of inventory, value of fees, and importance of good client service
- Can process all client financial transactions correctly
- Is able to explain practice's financial policies to clients
- Is able to explain a client invoice with an emphasis on value, not price

FIGURE 11.2 Level 2 Characteristics

A level 2 CSR will most likely have been with the practice at least six to nine months. This individual has a grasp of all the requirements of the level 1 CSR and additionally understands and displays the following characteristics and performs the following tasks.

General

- Welcomes and supports new team members; able to mentor new CSR hires
- Shows grace under pressure when working in stressful situations with difficult clients or team shortages
- Reflects positive practice cultural characteristics
- Openly communicates difficulties with supervisors

Communication

- Understands common parasites, zoonotic diseases, basic diagnostic testing methods, and symptoms of common medical problems
- Understands subtle communication clues such as tone of voice and body language
- Is able to calm clients during escalating situations
- Appropriately handles minor client complaints
- Is responsible for callbacks to clients after services, relaying doctor messages or follow-up on clients' complaints

Computer

- Accurately makes data entry corrections
- Prints end-of-day reports, reminders, and statements as directed
- Troubleshoots minor computer problems
- Understands computer backup process

Medical Records

- Assists in medical record auditing procedures
- Provides copies for clients as requested by the veterinary medical team
- Files or stores pet insurance documentation
- Responds to clients' requests for medical records

Operations

- Monitors reception area for violations of safety protocols and corrects them as necessary
- Is able to instruct new hires in general facility operations
- Understands functions of all veterinary personnel
- Has basic understanding of all veterinary medical functions in the practice: radiology, ultrasonography, surgery, pharmacy, etc.
- Orders office supplies

Financial

- Is able to make computer corrections as allowed
- Creates end-of-day report for the CSR team
- Monitors financial transactions of others
- Ensures appropriate change is available in the cash drawer

11

FIGURE 11.3 Level 3 Characteristics

A level 3 CSR will most likely have been with the practice for at least a year. This individual has a grasp of all the requirements of the level 1 and 2 CSRs and additionally understands and displays the following characteristics and performs the following tasks.

General

- Is an advocate for the practice
- Understands and relates the practice's philosophy and mission to teammates, clients, and other sources
- Is an example to other CSRs
- Adheres to practice policies
- Brings concerns from the CSR department to the supervisor
- Acts as a liaison to other departments in the practice

Communication

- Has veterinary knowledge: knows names and general use of common veterinary medications, is able to explain diagnostic testing to clients in basic terms, appropriately identifies emergency situations, advocates for best pet health care to clients
- Explains practice policies with aplomb during difficult client interactions
- Balances empathy with responsibility
- Is trusted with difficult communications, discussing CSR errors with clients, etc.

Computer

- Processes statements and end-of-month reports
- Troubleshoots computer problems and notifies IT personnel if necessary
- Troubleshoots software issues and is in contact with software provider
- Is responsible for security of backup procedures
- Is responsible for generation of and follow-through on reports such as reminders, statements, end-of-month, productivity, etc.

Medical Records

- Performs and reports on medical record auditing procedures
- Designs new medical record procedures in conjunction with medical team members
- Monitors and reports on new clients and referral sources

Operations

- Helps create operations policy when CSR operations are involved
- Trains new hires in general operations features that affect CSRs
- Can provide tours of the facility and overview of medical departments
- Monitors and reports on client complaint frequency and referral sources

Financial

- Closes financial transactions
- May make deposits
- Responsible for data entry and follow-up on bad checks and collection
- Advises other CSRs on practice financial policies

As you can see from the variety of tasks and responsibilities included for these three levels, the position of the CSR in our practice has growth potential. If you are already at the level 2 or 3 stage, please review the SOPs in this manual, looking for opportunities for growth and goal-setting. Remember that we want you to be with our practice for a long time and to continue to grow in the career path you've chosen.

AAHA Client Service Protocols

AHA is an organization that accredits veterinary hospitals. Practices desiring to be AAHA-accredited must pass a strenuous evaluation based on more than 900 veterinary standards. Among those standards are several written protocols affecting all areas of the practice, including the front office. The following are some of the client service protocols addressed in the current standards that contain helpful information for all practices.

APPEARANCE

No matter how you look at it, appearance helps make or break a first impression. Because we rely on first impressions as a relationship builder in our practice, we will always work to create a positive first impression by dressing and acting appropriately. The practice should have a written protocol that details practice team members' appearance, with emphasis on the impact of client trust and communication.

The purpose of creating this protocol is to maintain a professional appearance and attitude in order to make a positive impression on clients. This protocol should also be mentioned in the practice handbook and taught to all incoming personnel. It will be reinforced with individual team members as necessary. Team members should be self-regulating under the guidelines of this protocol. Supervisors and ultimately the hospital management should provide input to a team member as necessary.

COMMUNICATION

The practice should have a written client communication protocol that details how topics such as diagnosis, prognosis, therapeutic plans, cost of services, and follow-up are communicated to clients.

This protocol is meant to enhance a practice's ability to express the quality of service offered and to minimize the risk of misunderstanding between clients and the practice. This protocol should be part of the training program and should be reviewed and developed as practice needs change.

Every team member who comes into contact with our clientele must know and understand her role in the client communication process. She must demonstrate good communication skills across the responsibilities of her position at all times in order to progress at our practice. Team members' communication abilities are reviewed by their direct supervisor and the hospital management staff. Communication responsibilities include but are not limited to the following:

- An introduction to the practice
- On appointment
- Continuing communication
- Emergency
- Financial information
- Estimates
- Medical information (usually communicated by a member of the medical team)

CONFLICT IN CLIENT SERVICE

The practice should use a written client conflict protocol to help effectively address distraught and angry clients, including topics such as who will handle client communications and how the conflict and follow-up will be addressed.

It is important to educate the practice team member on how to deal with clients when a difficult situation arises. Team member training should be initiated at the time of hiring, and education should be completed and the knowledge foundation approved before direct contact with clients. The team member's direct supervisor and ultimately the management team are responsible for implementation of this protocol.

Client conflict may develop over various issues that may dictate how a team member will diffuse the situation. Typical examples are included here; however, the team must realize that resolution of client conflict may follow any iteration of the described protocols:

- Financial
- Medical
- Phone

If a client becomes verbally abusive and will not calm down when asked, team members should excuse themselves from the client's presence and seek the help of management.

If a team member feels threatened, she should ask for help immediately. If there is no one around to help, she should exit the area, seek help, and, if necessary, call the police.

FORMS

The practice should use a written forms protocol that includes how a form is reproduced (e.g., copied, printed, or electronic format) to maintain a clean, crisp professional appearance.

The purpose of creating this protocol is to ensure that the practice has professionally prepared and reproduced forms to promote the efficient operation of the practice and project the desired image. The information should be presented to new trainees and reviewed at least annually. Supervisors and the management team are responsible for managing implementation of the protocol.

PRACTICE PHILOSPHIES

Practice philosophy and protocols regarding topics such as how clients and patients are greeted, promptness of service, and payment options should be detailed in writing.

The purpose of this protocol is to enhance the consistency of communication, client trust, and the value of client service in the practice. It should be discussed during team member training for all areas of the practice. Supervisors and hospital management are responsible for seeing that team members understand and adhere to its principles.

PROFESSIONAL CONDUCT

The practice should use a written protocol for professional conduct, such as the following:

- Respect for other practice team members
- Respect for clients
- Respect for animals (alive or deceased)
- Conduct in the presence of clients
- Body language
- Verbal and written communication

The purpose of creating this protocol is to ensure that the practice team accepts responsibility for and demonstrates a uniform and high level of professional conduct, ethics, and behavior. This code of conduct will be practiced at all times in the hospital.

New team members will be trained to this high level of conduct and team members will be held accountable for any lapses. Ultimate responsibility for enforcing this protocol lies with the management.

This policy of professional conduct should be explained at the interview and taught during the initial on-boarding of new team members. This protocol should be reviewed with the entire team as necessary and at the annual practice review.

APPENDIX A
COMMON VETERINARY ABBREVIATIONS

Abbreviation	Definition
A	
Ab	Antibodies
Abd	Abdomen
Abx	Antibiotics
Ace	Acepromazine
ACL	Anterior cruciate ligament
ACTH	Adrenocorticotropic hormone
ACTH Stim	ACTH stimulation test
AD	*Auris dextra*, right ear
Ad lib	*Ad libitum*, at (one's) pleasure
ADR	Ain't doing right
ALP	Alkaline phosphatase
ALT	Alanine aminotransferase (*formerly* SGPT)
Anes	Anesthesia
Ant	Anterior
AP	Anterioposterior
Appt	Appointment
AS	*Auris sinistra*, left ear
AST	Aspartate aminotransferase (*formerly* SGOT)
AU	*Auris utraque*, both ears
B	
BAR	Bright, alert, responsive
BCS	Body condition score
BG	Blood glucose
bid	*Bis in die*, twice a day
BP	Blood pressure
BPM	Beats per minute
BUN	Blood urea nitrogen
BW	Body weight
Bx	Biopsy

C

CaOx .... Calcium oxalate

cap(s) .... Capsule(s)

CBC .... Complete blood cell count

Chem .... Chemistry panel

CHF .... Congestive heart failure

CNS .... Central nervous system

CPR .... Cardiopulmonary resuscitation

Creat .... Creatinine

CRI .... Constant rate infusion

CRT .... Capillary refill time

C/S .... Coughing/sneezing

C&S .... Culture and sensitivity

D

D5W .... 5% dextrose in water

DA2PP .... Distemper, adenovirus type 2, parainfluenza, parvovirus

DA2PPL .... Distemper, adenovirus type 2, parainfluenza, parvovirus, leptospirosis

DDx .... Differential diagnosis

DDz .... Dental disease

Derm .... Dermatology

Disp .... Dispensed

DJD................. Degenerative joint disease

DKA .... Diabetic ketoacidosis

dl .... Deciliter

DM .... Diabetes mellitus

DV.................. Dorsoventral

Dx .... Diagnosis

Dz .... Disease

E

ECC.................. Emergency and critical care

ECG .... Electrocardiogram (*see* EKG)

E Collar .... Elizabethan collar

EKG .... Electrocardiogram (*see* ECG)

ET .... Endotracheal tube

Euth .... Euthanize (*see* PTS)

F

FAD .... Flea allergy dermatitis
FB .... Foreign body
FeL .... Feline
FeLV................ Feline leukemia virus
FIP .... Feline infectious peritonitis
FIV .... Feline immunodeficiency virus
FLUTD .... Feline lower urinary tract disease
FNA .... Fine needle aspirate
FS .... Spayed female
fT_4ED............... Free T_4 by equilibrium dialysis
FUO .... Fever of unknown origin
FUS .... Feline urologic syndrome
FVRCP .... Feline viral rhinotracheitis, calicivirus,
                panleukopenia
Fx .... Fracture

G

GDV................ Gastric dilatation-volvulus
GI................... Gastrointestinal
Glu .... Glucose

H

HBC .... Hit by car
HC.................. Health certificate
HCT .... Hematocrit
H/L .... Heart and lungs
HPF .... High-power field
HR.................. Heart rate
HW .... Heartworm
HWDz .... Heartworm disease
HWT .... Heartworm test
Hx .... History

I

IBD................. Inflammatory bowel disease
IM .... Intramuscular
IN................... Intranasal
Inj .... Injection, injectable
IV................... Intravenous

IV Cath .... Intravenous catheter
IVDD................ Intervertebral disk disease

J

Jt .... Joint

K

K9 .... Canine
kcal .... Kilocalorie
Ket/Val .... Ketamine and valium
kg .... Kilogram

L

l .... Liter
Lat .... Lateral
lb .... Pound
LF................... Left front
LM .... Left message
LN.................. Lymph node(s)
LPF .... Low-power field
LR .... Left rear
LRS .... Lactated Ringer's solution

M

M .... Medial
mEq .... Milliequivalent
mg .... Milligram
ml .... Milliliter
MM .... Mucous membranes
MN .... Neutered male

N

NC.................. No change
Neg .... Negative
Neuro .... Neurology, neurological
NPL .... No palpable lesions
NPO................ Nothing *per os*, nothing by mouth
NSAID .... Nonsteroidal anti-inflammatory drug
NSF................. No significant findings

O

O_2 .... Oxygen
OA .... Osteoarthritis

OD....................*Oculus dexter*, right eye

OHE..................Ovariohysterectomy

O/P ....Ova and parasites

Ophtho..............Ophthalmology

OS....................*Oculus sinister*, left eye

OTC..................Over the counter

OU ....*Oculus uterque*, both eyes

P

PCV ....Packed cell volume

PE ....Physical examination

Pl ....Plantar

PLR...................Pupillary light response

PO....................*Per os*, by mouth

Pos ....Positive

PostOp ....Postoperative

Pred ....Prednisone

PreOp ....Preoperative

prn ....*Pro re nata*, as needed

PTS ....Put to sleep (*see* Euth)

PU/PD ....Polyuria and polydipsia

Px ....Prognosis

Q

q......................*Quaque*, every (*as in* q 2 h—every two hours)

QAR.................Quiet, alert, responsive

qod ....Every other day

R

Rads.................Radiographs (*see* Xray)

RBC ....Red blood cell

RF ....Right front

RO....................Rule out

RR....................Right rear

RTG ....Ready to go (home)

Rx ....Prescription, prescribed

S

SC ....Subcutaneous (*see* SQ)

SG ....Specific gravity

sid ....*Semel in die*, once a day

Sig .... Instructions on prescription label

SOAP .... Subjective, objective, assessment, plan

SQ .... Subcutaneous (*see* SC)

SR .... Suture removal

Sx .... Surgery

T

T_4 .... Tetraiodothyronine, thyroxine

tab(s) .... Tablet(s)

tid .... Ter in die, three times a day

TNTC................ Too numerous to count

TPR.................. Temperature, pulse, respiration

Tx .... Treatment

U

UA .... Urinalysis

URI.................... Upper respiratory infection

URT .... Upper respiratory tract

US .... Ultrasound

USG .... Urine specific gravity

UTI.................... Urinary tract infection

V

Vacc .... Vaccination (*see* Vx)

VD.................... Ventrodorsal

V/D.................... Vomiting and diarrhea

Vx .... Vaccination (*see* Vacc)

W

WBC .... White blood cell count

WNL .... Within normal limits

Wt.................... Weight

X

Xray .... Radiograph (*see* Rads)

APPENDIX B
MANAGER'S APPENDIX

As noted in the Introduction, there are areas of the text that may be modified to the specifics of your practice. If you want to customize this text, use this section of the book to help you. Each chapter that has sections requiring modification is listed here with instructions on how to create the customization. SOPs and other sections that you may want to customize are included on the CD that accompanies this book, allowing you to easily make the necessary changes. But first let's begin with an overview of writing an SOP.

HOW TO WRITE AN SOP

An SOP is a document that details all the steps and activities of a process in your practice. Following an SOP helps create uniformity and improve efficiency and quality of service across the team.

SOPs can be created for many of the procedures in your practice. Most tasks have a *best* procedural method, that is, a method that when followed creates the best outcome. For example, veterinarians follow surgical SOPs when performing surgeries recommending the use of certain types of techniques and materials. Veterinary technicians follow SOPs when using blood machines to perform blood analysis, and CSRs use SOPs for running charges on a credit card machine. Any multistep procedure or task that would benefit from standardized execution may be a good candidate for an SOP.

Creating SOPs is not difficult for most managers. It is time-consuming, but you can enlist the help of your team members who perform these tasks every day. A good way to start is to ask the individuals who perform the task frequently to write down, in numbered steps, what it takes to accomplish the task. This endeavor serves two purposes: It gives you a compilation of the steps necessary to complete the task, and it lets you know the various methods individual team members are using to perform the task. You may be surprised by the procedures your team is using to complete any one task!

When writing your SOP, be specific and clear in your instructions. Break the task down into small steps and think of how new team members, who know nothing about your practice, will follow your instructions. Your SOP for scheduling an appointment might begin by saying, "Open the appointment scheduler on the computer by clicking on the icon that looks like a book." Or, if you do your computer training early in a new team member's experience, you might start by saying, "With the appointment scheduler open on the computer, find the time slot requested by the client." Or perhaps you will have everyone trained on the computer before they are allowed to schedule appointments, so you want to begin by saying, "Our practice schedules appointments in fifteen-minute, thirty-minute, forty-five-minute, and one-hour increments. Fifteen-minute time slots are used for . . . ." Much of the specifics of your SOPs will depend on your practice's training methodology.

With the SOP created, ask a team member to try to complete the task, following only the directions in the SOP. This will help you determine any weaknesses in your SOP. Once it is created, if changes have been made to the "way in which we have always done it," you will need to do some retraining with your current team.

Although it is not difficult to create an SOP, it can be difficult to get everyone to adhere to it. The task is made easier if you can show the team why the standard process helps the patient, the client, the team member, and the practice. When evaluating the success of your SOP and training the team, remember that your team will fall back on the method that works for them. People, fairly naturally, look for shortcuts. If these shortcuts don't hurt the power of the SOP, try incorporating them. It will save you some headaches and empower your team. If the change *does* hurt the power of the SOP, weakening it or creating confusion, sit down with the individual who is circumventing your method and help him understand the consequences of his actions, and how they affect patient care and the practice. Ask and require him to conform to the SOP.

SOPs need to be reviewed frequently. New technology, new personnel, new products, and even facility changes can affect the processes used within a practice. Your SOP may need to change when any of these changes takes place. Don't wait to—and don't be afraid to—change your SOPs as frequently as necessary so that they remain pertinent to your practice.

INTRODUCTION

Everything starts with a good introduction. Making a strong connection with your new CSRs will facilitate learning and your ability to coach and mentor them as they progress. Don't be afraid, as you customize this portion of the text, to let the personality of your practice show through. Tell your new team members some of the history of your practice and give them a big welcome as they find their place on your team.

The Process of On-boarding

The on-boarding process may vary somewhat with the specific organizational structure and procedures of your practice. All these steps take place after the hiring process, although aspects of them (review of the job description, for instance) may also be used during the hiring process.

1. **New hire orientation.** This should be a one-on-one overview of basic practice information. It may be conducted by a member of your human resources team but can be a good bonding experience for the new team member to a direct supervisor or mentoring teammate. It will include the following:

    a. Introduction to the staff.

    b. Facility design, use, and location of various functions. Stress how these functions work together as a whole to reach the practice's goals.

    c. Basic safety information, including evacuation, fire extinguisher location, location of MSDS information, etc.

    d. Basic everyday working procedures, including reporting to work and leaving, work routines, location and assignment of lockers, location of the lunch room, designated parking, etc.

2. **Review the practice's core values, mission, and vision.** Hopefully these were introduced during the hiring process. Coming back to them now and during the training process will help focus your new hires on the foundational practice beliefs and how their responsibilities tie into the global mission.

3. **Review of job description in detail.** Sit down with the new hires and go back over their responsibilities. Urge them to ask questions if anything seems unclear. Make a point of noting their responsibilities in the process and what they must be able to do after their training to fulfill the job description.

4. **Introduction to the training timeline and assigned mentors.** It is important to have trained mentors to reach out to new team members and help them acclimate to the new practice. Mentors should be chosen from the tenured team for their social skills as well as their technical skills. New hires will learn much more than technical skills from their mentors. They will learn about how things work in your practice. As a manager you need to know that mentors will be presenting the appropriate picture of your practice culture. This meeting should be an opportunity for new hires to dig deeper into what will be required of them during training.

5. **The training process.** Schedule frequent reviews and opportunities for supervisors to check in and be sure progress is on track. Monitor their progress.

6. **Review.** As necessary, take a step back to any section of this process and review the information that has already been provided. It may be necessary to recall parts of the orientation day or sections of the job description as you move through training in order for new hires to fully grasp their responsibilities.

To the New Team Member

It is important to provide new team members with accurate information about your hospital's history. This information will help them understand the culture and the practice's daily mission. You can often get this information from your practice website or employee handbook. It can be brief but should provide a foundation of understanding your practice. It might look something like this:

> *Our veterinary practice began in 2007 when Dr. Megan Smith opened this facility. Dr. Smith is a graduate of The Ohio State University, where she studied from 1999 to 2002. She was a pet lover from an early age, owning her first kitten by the time she was six, and participated in 4-H and various animal-related clubs and associations. Her team consists of several certified veterinary technicians and dedicated support team members. We are unified by the desire to provide the highest-quality care offered in northeastern Pennsylvania. The practice offers pet health care to pocket pets, cats, and dogs and is accredited through the American Animal Hospital Association.*

Welcome Aboard!

This would be a great place to customize the text with information about your practice's organizational structure and the names of particular individuals who will be supervising new team members. The text includes a place to insert the name of a CSR's primary supervisor and an organizational chart. The organizational chart is like a road map to the hierarchy of your practice and can be very helpful in orienting the new team member to the role played by the specific team members.

CHAPTER 1

This chapter continues your introduction to new team members but also helps them understand your expectations for them during their time with your practice.

Our Hospital's Core Values, Mission, and Vision

These three tenets of your practice can be fundamental to the development of your practice culture. They can be the very basis of every management decision you make and will guide your team when they must make decisions "on the go." Begin by creating a core value list. This may be done in conjunction with your management group and perhaps your entire team. It should consist of a list of three to five items that you believe are *bottom-line* decision makers for your management group and that you wish to see promulgated throughout your team.

You must live by these as well as express them in front of your team, so be careful to choose items that ring true for you. They might consist of the following: honesty, as expressed by telling the truth; responsibility, as expressed by doing what you say you will do. I suggest the clarifying statements (e.g., "as expressed by") to provide examples and promote understanding of the terms. This is a great exercise for a retreat or extended team meeting.

The practice's mission statement will grow from the core value list. Create a statement that reflects what you want to be doing each day. Ideally, the statement will be short enough that team members can commit it to heart and use it as their "guiding light" during stressful moments. For example, if your mission statement includes the statement: "We will create a positive client experience for each pet's visit," your CSRs can fall back on that when they are being worn thin by a difficult client.

The vision statement arises from a compilation of thoughts about the practice's position in a more global picture. How would you want the practice to be described on its twenty-fifth or fiftieth anniversary of service to the community? What do you hope to be in the future?

The practice's core values might be listed in this manner:

Quality care, as expressed in offering cutting-edge medical procedures in a caring manner. We will care for each pet as a precious loved one.

Responsibility, as expressed as individuals doing what they have said they will do in a timely manner. We are responsible to our clients, their pets, and each other.

Communication, as expressed by being thorough, truthful, and caring in all our communications. We understand the value of providing accurate information in a manner appropriate to the individual with whom we are communicating. We endeavor to reach out to each person in a caring manner.

Respect, as expressed by the way we speak to and treat every person and pet. Every person is entitled to his or her own opinion and is responsible for expressing that opinion in an appropriate manner.

Teamwork, as expressed by the way we work together. We believe that we are a stronger organization when we work together. We will be better able to meet the challenges of our profession by relying on each other.

A vision statement might read something like the following:

Our vision is to have an acclaimed veterinary practice, known for its quality medical care, advanced services, and caring attitude. We want to be the veterinary practice of choice for our region, the place to which people bring their pets with confidence and about which they tell their friends.

Finally, a mission statement might read something like the following:

We are veterinary professionals dedicated to providing compassionate, quality pet care in a manner that reflects our responsibility to those that visit our practice and to each other. We will be financially responsible with our resources, innovative in our approach to veterinary medicine, and caring in all that we do.

Your Job Description

Most practices have a CSR job description. The purpose of this section is to refocus new team members on the overall picture of their place in the practice and then draw attention to the individual tasks that are required of them. In doing so, we hope to instill a deeper understanding of the value of what they do each day.

If you have not yet created a job description, you can seek guidance from the following example (Figure A.1) or look for information in another publication. It may be helpful to ask your established CSRs to create a list of what they do each day and use it to fashion your list of CSR duties and tasks.

Your Training Schedule

In this section, you should break down your training tasks into associated areas and provide your new team members with a format for becoming competent in these tasks (see Figure A.2). You may wish to be more or less detailed, lengthening or shortening the time frame as it fits your practice. The point is to affirm your expectations with your new team members and give them some idea of how quickly they are required to become proficient in their task responsibilities. You must remember that individuals learn by different methods and at different speeds. Your timetable should be somewhat flexible. Assess each new team member to determine whether he or she will do better by learning all tasks of a certain type at one time or by following a client through the process of checking in, the appointment, and checking out. The text includes an outline of a timeline for anywhere from one week to three months. You may wish to continue this to include up to a year of training. You will want to fill in the dates as applicable. In addition to the training schedule listed in Chapter 1, a CSR's secondary responsibilities might include items from the following list or other duties as defined by your practice:

FIGURE A.1 Job Description

ANYTOWN VETERINARY HOSPITAL
JOB DESCRIPTION

Job Title: Client service representative
Reports to: Client service supervisor and practice manager
Schedule: Varies according to business needs, but may include weekends, evenings, and holidays; approximately forty hours per week

Summary
The CSR's goal is to help the practice team provide the best in client and patient care and to improve efficiency and team effectiveness by constantly working to improve his or her personal level of competency and the practice's efficiency. CSRs should be professional, reliable, honest, civil, cheerful, and enthusiastic; have a strong work ethic; and have a high level of empathy for suffering pets and people. Any person(s) working in this position will play an essential role in upholding the mission of the practice, as described in the following.

Major Goals
- To be efficient, pleasant, courteous, caring, and helpful to all clients and coworkers under all conditions and at all times
- To provide the best service to all clientele
- To support the overall mission of the practice to provide advanced quality veterinary care for pets and empathetic, compassionate care to their owners while understanding and representing the needs of the team and the practice

Essential Duties and Responsibilities
- Greet and assist clients in a professional and courteous manner.
- Promptly answer and direct incoming calls.
- Accurately input data in the computer.
- Accurately process client transactions.
- Support and empathize with clients; always act in a caring manner.
- Assist in organizing and cleaning the client service area.
- Properly maintain medical records.
- Uphold the practice's mission, vision, and core values.
- Other essential tasks as assigned.

Education, Experience, and Qualifications
The candidate must have a high school diploma or the equivalent. Past veterinary experience is helpful. Customer service experience is essential. The individual must be able to work independently on projects in a team environment.

The candidate must have good verbal and written communication skills, understand basic telephone etiquette, and work in an organized manner. Attention to detail is required. The candidate

continues >>

FIGURE A.1 Job Description, continued

must have basic mathematical skills and handle currency correctly: making change, entering payments into the computer, and finalizing end-of-day procedures. The candidate must be able to define problems, collect data, establish facts, and draw valid conclusions in client care situations. Understanding and use of computer and other electronic equipment are essential. Familiarity with additional computer programs such as Word and Excel is helpful.

Work Environment
The veterinary practice may be noisy at times. You will be required to be able to lift forty pounds. There are hazardous chemicals present within the facility, and radiographic equipment is used on the premises. You will be required to sit, stand, and move about frequently.

The above job description is not an all-inclusive list of duties. Your supervisor or another member of the practice team may at times assign duties other than those mentioned here.

Team Member Signature: _____   Date: _____
Client Service Supervisor Signature: _____   Date: _____

Secondary Responsibilities

1. **Marketing opportunities.** Attend local school career days, participate in dog walks, or work with the emergency disaster relief organization to establish rescue guidelines.
2. **Team-building opportunities.** Help plan the Christmas party or lead a topical discussion at the team meeting, participate in a grief counseling program, etc.
3. **Cross-training opportunities.** Become familiar with the tasks associated with another job position within the practice, learn to hold pets for examination, process a medication refill, or do general housekeeping chores.

How You Will Be Evaluated

Included here are very basic performance review procedures, including a sample form. Your practice may use a similar format but at different times, or may use a completely different format. Formal evaluations are recommended. It is important to let the new team member know what to expect as a review of his or her work in the coming months.

FIGURE A.2 Client Service Representative Performance Appraisal

ANYTOWN VETERINARY HOSPITAL
CLIENT SERVICE REPRESENTATIVE PERFORMANCE APPRAISAL

Name: _____   **Date:** _____

Major goals: The CSR's primary responsibilities revolve around creating a good client experience and presenting a professional image to the public. Several specific skills that enhance an individual's ability to fulfill these responsibilities are evaluated here.

Please use the following rating system:
5 = Highly effective   4 = Effective   3 = Average   2 = Needs improvement   1 = Poor   n/a = Not applicable

Essential Duties and Responsibilities:

Greets clients promptly and has a warm, friendly manner.	5	4	3	2	1	n/a
Demonstrates good phone etiquette by providing appropriate identifying information, speaking clearly, and efficiently addressing callers' needs.	5	4	3	2	1	n/a
Demonstrates efficient work habits, using time wisely and addressing clients' needs first.	5	4	3	2	1	n/a
Demonstrates ability to reason through complex situations and apply good judgment.	5	4	3	2	1	n/a
Properly organizes and cleans work area and client reception area.	5	4	3	2	1	n/a
Understands and follows practice protocols regarding financial transactions.	5	4	3	2	1	n/a
Clearly explains to clients all practice protocols involving financial transactions.	5	4	3	2	1	n/a
Properly enters data into computer, creating accurate computer records.	5	4	3	2	1	n/a
Schedules appointments with the needs of both the practice and the client in mind.	5	4	3	2	1	n/a
Empathetically interacts with distraught or difficult clients.	5	4	3	2	1	n/a
Works well with teammates: Encourages others, offers constructive comments, and accepts the feedback of others.	5	4	3	2	1	n/a
Demonstrates acceptable level of veterinary knowledge: familiar with common terms, diagnostic testing, treatments, and OTC prescription medications.	5	4	3	2	1	n/a
Demonstrates understanding of and alignment with the practice's core values, mission statement, and vision statements.	5	4	3	2	1	n/a

Areas of particular strength:
_____

Areas of opportunity:
_____

Additional information for review:
_____

Future goals, including accomplishment dates:
_____

Employee feedback on evaluation:
_____

Team Member Signature: _____   Date: _____
Reviewer Name: _____
Reviewer Signature: _____   Date: _____

CHAPTER 2

This chapter includes pieces of information that will help your new CSR become more familiar with the terminology of everyday life in the veterinary practice. It describes job titles, basic terminology, and terminology related to specific veterinary situations.

Preventive Care

Because much preventive care is based on the patient's stage of life, many practices coordinate their care with a patient's age. You may want to customize the life-stage protocols suggested below for use in your practice. It will be helpful for your new team members to know what happens at each stage. Your protocols may include the following:

- **Puppy and kitten visits.** This visit may include vaccination schedules, fecal testing and routine deworming, and procedures such as heartworm testing and spaying or neutering. There are convenient quick tests available for use in detecting diseases that may be present but not causing immediate symptoms, such as feline leukemia virus (FeLV) and feline immunodeficiency virus (FIV).

- **Dogs and cats older than six years of age.** Many practices use routine diagnostic testing for animals older than six. If your practice does so, it will be helpful for your new team members to become familiar with those diagnostics. This list may include items such as routine CBC and chest Xrays in addition to the recommended vaccine schedule and fecal sampling. Discussion of dietary needs, weight management, and oral care should also be included. There may even be particular diagnostic testing routines that your veterinarians prefer for pets who have reached the last years of their lives, such as more frequent blood work for early recognition of kidney disease.

The Importance of Vaccinations

Recommendations for vaccination schedules have varied with advancements in the veterinary profession. Your veterinarian will undoubtedly have a preferred timeline. Following is a suggested schedule based on the AAHA and AAFP (American Association of Feline Practitioners) Canine and Feline Vaccination Guidelines.

- Canine
  - » Distemper combination (DA2PP) should be started at six to eight weeks; booster every three to four weeks until twenty weeks of age. This vaccination will be good for a year and can be administered to the adult dog every three years after that.
  - » Bordetella and parainfluenza (intranasal) should be started at between three and six weeks for at-risk dogs, with a booster in two to four weeks, and then again at six months to one year, depending on the patient's risk of exposure. For adult dogs, they may be administered every six months to a year, depending on risk.

» In our area, Lyme vaccination should begin in puppies at nine weeks of age, with a booster in two to three weeks. The vaccine lasts for a year, and adults should be revaccinated yearly.

» Leptospirosis vaccination should be administered at twelve weeks for at-risk dogs, with a booster in three to four weeks; it is good for a year. Adults should be vaccinated yearly.

» Rabies vaccination should be given at twelve weeks, and this first vaccination is good for a year. Three-year vaccines are available and can be administered to adult dogs.

- Feline
  » Feline distemper combination (FVRCP) should be given to kittens at six weeks, with a booster every three to four weeks until sixteen weeks of age. The vaccination lasts for a year and should be administered to adult cats every three years thereafter.

  » FeLV vaccination can be given to kittens at between eight and ten weeks, with a booster once in three to four weeks; it is good for a year. Adult cats who received the vaccine as a kitten should be revaccinated every three years.

  » Rabies vaccination should be administered to kittens at twelve weeks. The vaccination is good for a year, and cats should be revaccinated at that time and then either yearly or every three years, depending on the type of vaccine preferred by the practice.

Client Education

It takes a long time for a new CSR to become familiar with the various client education materials available in your practice. Ask a tenured team member to collect samples of each pamphlet or brochure you routinely use and create a list of the various titles. These materials can be placed in your training notebooks for review by new team members.

Common Illnesses or Conditions

You may want to add or subtract from the information provided here. Perhaps there are diseases or pet problems that are prevalent in your region and are of particular importance to your new team member.

Common Diagnostic Procedures

Every practice uses a slightly different array of diagnostic equipment. Your new team member will need to become familiar with these items and their functions as quickly as possible. You can customize this section to the particulars of your practice by adding a list of the equipment you have and its general functions. You may want to include the full list so your employees will be aware of other diagnostic equipment available in the veterinary world. You can recruit a member of your technical team to help create this list, or you can review your files for equipment purchases. When describing the function, remember that your new CSR will not need to know how the machine works but just the basic description of its medical function. This list should include laboratory, imaging, and monitoring equipment.

Sample: Our practice uses a _____ ultrasonography unit and our doctors interpret the images themselves or send them out to be interpreted by a specialist.

Hospitalization

Your practice may or may not offer overnight hospitalization. If you do, the services offered may vary. Some hospitals have veterinarians on staff overnight, others have technical team members, and still others have no one on the premises. Clients may be nervous about their pet staying in your hospital, and a CSR who is knowledgeable about your hospitalization protocols will be a great help in soothing their nerves. Make sure your new team members are provided with a list of what happens to the hospitalized pet.

Surgical Procedures

You may want to create a customized list of the surgical procedures offered by your practice and the measures used by your surgical team to protect their patients.

CHAPTER 3

Although the basic principles of good client service ring true throughout the industry, each veterinary practice has specific challenges dependent on the current culture and the individuals who work there. You may have particular challenges you want to address and for which your practice has created or will want to create SOPs. The SOPs for this chapter are customizable.

CHAPTER 4

This chapter presents general information about good telephone etiquette and the importance of gathering the appropriate information from a caller. Many of the sections of this chapter may need to be customized to fit your practice.

Using Our Telephone System

This section must be customized for your practice to be helpful to the new CSR. It should include how your telephone system operates and whether there is an extension for medication refills, for emergencies, and for scheduling appointments. Or do all the calls come into a central line, and the CSR directs them from that point?

The SOPs for this chapter are all customizable.

CHAPTER 5

The most important information in this chapter is the practice's philosophy of appointment scheduling. It has been presented to new CSRs as a way of balancing the needs of the client and the needs of the practice. Helping them understand their responsibilities to both sides of this delicate balance will give them a strong foundation for decision making when they are scheduling clients. All appointment processes should be modified for your practice.

In this chapter, CSRs also learn about entering new client information into the computer. Veterinary practices usually train new team members verbally on how their computer system operates. One individual trains another, and there is little, if any, documentation of how to perform integral tasks. This can create various methods for completing a single task and typically results in lack of standardization. Written documentation of a how-to process increases the slope of the learning curve and provides security to new team members as they assimilate the multitude of information we heap on them in their first thirty days of employment.

Ask a competent CSR to create a how-to list of protocols for your practice's software, collect a series of the software's webinars (many systems have a downloadable format on their website), or in some other fashion give your new CSR information on the basic tasks he or she will have to perform.

This process should be completed for every standard software task for which the CSR will be responsible. Creating this bullet-pointed SOP will ensure that new team members are getting all the information they need to create consistently accurate data. Taking these few moments during the impressionable training period will instill good habits for the future.

The SOPs for this chapter are customizable.

CHAPTER 6

This chapter starts with a review of the importance of and proper method for greeting a client. Appointments are such an integral part of your practice's success that it is appropriate to present concepts regarding appointments in two chapters of the text. Although your practice's process of checking in and checking out may vary from the text in detail, the general flow will most likely be similar.

The SOPs for this chapter are customizable.

CHAPTER 7

Your practice may have marketing initiatives that require action by your CSR. Maybe the reminder cards are managed by this individual, or maybe you have particular promotions such as preventive health care plans that the CSR will offer your clients. These situations have not been addressed in the general text and may be added by you during customization. The SOPs for this chapter are customizable.

CHAPTER 8

Every practice struggles to some degree to collect payment from clients. Your new CSR needs to understand the value of your practice's services, at least some facts about the cost to offer those services, and how to talk to clients about payment. While the SOPs may need to be modified in this chapter for the particulars of your practice, the philosophies expressed will hold true. The SOPs for this chapter are customizable.

CHAPTER 9

As you know, the patient's medical record is a legal document and every practice team member should understand the implications of that statement. This chapter is designed to give new CSRs an understanding of their part in recording information in this document. It touches on the essentials of medical record keeping and their responsibilities. The SOPs for this chapter are customizable.

CHAPTER 10

This chapter is a general overview of safety for the new CSR and will provide a good introduction to your practice's safety training process. It is not an exhaustive safety training program. The SOP is customizable.

CHAPTER 11

New CSRs will progress through the levels of training and ability at varying rates. You will need to evaluate them on a regular basis by reviewing both the tasks they are able to complete and their assimilation of your culture and practice philosophies. These characteristics are general and need to be modified to fit your practice. The tasks associated with the characteristics should be itemized and presented to team members as they move through the levels. You may want to ask a CSR you identify as currently representing a particular level in your practice to help you create the list of tasks associated with performing at that level.

ENDNOTES

1   The Myers & Briggs Foundation, http://www.myersbriggs.org (accessed November 30, 2012).

2   Discprofile, http://www.discprofile.com (accessed November 30, 2012).

3   American Veterinary Medical History Society, http://www.avmhs.org/Welcome, home page.

4   American Veterinary Medical Association, "Human-Animal Bond," *Reference Guides*, https://www.avma.org/KB/Resources/Reference/human-animal-bond/Pages/Human-Animal-Bond-AVMA.aspx (accessed November 26, 2012).

5   *The Merriam-Webster Dictionary* (Springfield, MA: Merriam Webster, Inc., 2005).

6   American Veterinary Medical Association, "Model Veterinary Practice Act," *Policies*, https://www.avma.org/KB/Policies/Pages/Model-Veterinary-Practice-Act.aspx.

7   *Merriam-Webster's Collegiate Dictionary* (Springfield, Massachusetts: Merriam-Webster, Inc., 1995), 214.

8   Scott McKain, *All Business Is Show Business* (Nashville, Tennessee: Rutledge Hill Press, 2002): 18.

9   S. E. G. Lea and P. Webley, "Money as Tool, Money as Drug: The Biological Psychology of a Strong Incentive," *Behavioral and Brain Sciences* 29, 2, (2006): 161–209.

10 Laurel Lagoni, MS, and Dana Durrance, MA. *Connecting with Clients*, Second Edition (Lakewood, Colorado: AAHA Press, 2010): 57.

11 Ibid., 57.

12 Sandra Blakeslee, "Cells That Read Minds," *New York Times*, January 10, 2006.

13 Humane Society of the United States, "Coping with the Death of Your Pet," *Animal Care Community Resources*, http://www.humanesociety.org/animals/resources/tips/coping_with_pet_death (accessed November 26, 2012).

14 Helpguide.org, "Supporting a Grieving Person," *Grief & Loss Help Guide*, http://www.helpguide.org/mental/helping_grieving.htm (accessed November 26, 2012).

15 Laurel Lagoni, MS, and Dana Durrance, MA, *Connecting with Grieving Clients*, Second Edition (Lakewood, Colorado: AAHA Press, 2011): 18.

16 Marhsa L. Heinke, DVM, CPA, CVPM. *Practice Made Perfect*, Second Edition (Lakewood, Colorado: AAHA Press, 2012): 478.

17 Daniel Verdon, "Pet Owners Push Back," *DVM Newsmagazine*, September 1, 2011.

18 John Gottman and Nan Silver. *The Seven Principles for Making Marriage Work* (New York, New York: Three Rivers Press, 1999).

19   Marsha L. Heinke, DVM, CPA, CVPM. *Practice Made Perfect*, Second Edition (Lakewood, Colorado: AAHA Press, 2012): 488–509.

20   Robert Johnston, "The Determinants of Service Quality: Satisfiers and Dissatisfiers," *International Journal of Service: Industry Management* 6, 5 (1995): 53–71.

21   Graham Roberts-Phelps. *Companies Don't Succeed, People Do* (Abingdon, United Kingdom: Thorogood, 2000): 7.

FOR THE CSR

Adam, Cindy, PhD, MSW, *Communication Matters*, online course (Guelph, Ontario, Canada: LifeLearn Inc.).

American Animal Hospital Association, *Standard Abbreviations for Veterinary Medical Records*, Third Edition (Lakewood, Colorado: AAHA Press, 2010).

Grosdidier, Sheila, *Essentials of Client Service*, online course (Guelph, Ontario, Canada: LifeLearn Inc.).

Lagoni, Laurel, MS, and Dana Durrance, MA, *Connecting with Clients*, Second Edition (Lakewood, Colorado: AAHA Press, 2010).

Lagoni, Laurel, MS, and Dana Durrance, MA, *Connecting with Grieving Clients*, Second Edition (Lakewood, Colorado: AAHA Press, 2011).

Prendergast, Heather, BS, AS, RVT, CVPM, *Front Office Management for the Veterinary Team* (Philadelphia, Pennsylvania: WB Saunders, 2010).

FOR THE MANAGER

American Animal Hospital Association, "On-Hold Phone Script," *Promoting Our Accreditation*, www.aahanet.org/accreditation (accessed February 22, 2013).

Heinke, Marsha L., DVM, CPA, CVPM, *Practice Made Perfect*, Second Edition (Lakewood, Colorado: AAHA Press, 2012).

Smith, Carin A., DVM, *Client Satisfaction Pays*, Second Edition (Lakewood, Colorado: AAHA Press, 2009).

Wilson, James F., DVM, JD, and Karen Gendron, DVM, *Job Descriptions and Training Schedules* (Pennsylvania: Priority Press, 2005).

INDEX

W

Z